GUINEA PIG ZERO

An Anthology of the Journal For
Human Research Subjects

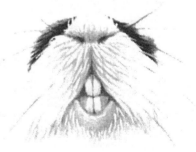

GUINEA PIG ZERO

AN ANTHOLOGY OF THE JOURNAL
FOR HUMAN RESEARCH SUBJECTS

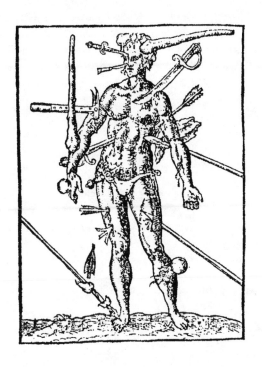

edited by
ROBERT HELMS

Garrett County Press

Garrett County Press, LLC
828 Royal St. #248
New Orleans, LA 70116
www.gcpress.com

This GCPress book printed on recycled, acid free paper.

Library of Congress Control Number: 2002104186
       1.Hospitals--Case Studies--Moral and ethical aspects.
       2.Medical ethics--history.
       3.Medical research--history.
ISBN: 1-891053-84-1

Garrett County Press first edition 2002

Random act of cover art by Jeremy Schulz
Inside illustrations by Dug
Cover and text design by Hac H. Le,
iCONiKLaSTique Design Klinik, LLC
www.iDKdesign.com

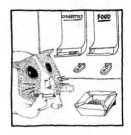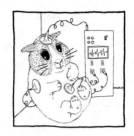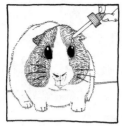

ILLUSTRATIONS BY DUG

INTRODUCTION

Before publishing the first issue of *Guinea Pig Zero* on May 1, 1996, I had been developing my skills in organized resistance in the workplace for several years. In 1990 I participated in student protest actions in support of the striking faculty at Temple University, and I then took a job as a field organizer, bringing new groups of (mostly health care) workers into union membership. From 1991-94, I spent a lot of time campaigning with Human Services personnel who cared for mentally retarded adults in far-flung suburban "group homes."

During those four years, I gained a knowledge of the problems of bringing together people who work for the same company but almost never meet one another. Any campaign for workers' rights will be difficult at best, but when the workers are scattered and isolated, it may seem downright impossible. In spite of the obstacles, I was able to lead a few hundred such people into union representation. From this experience I found that I could never again obey an arrogant boss who exploits and verbally abuses his or her employees. I now instinctively look for ways to wipe the filthy smirks off their faces. All this experience served me well after I left the union job, stopped wearing a tie, and found work as a freelance human guinea pig.

When I rent my healthy body to medical science, I am the temporary employee of a research team, paid as a contractor for each job. I do my bleeding, pissing work in a blurry area between patient and subject. This blurry area has made for intense public debate, and the questions relating to the guinea pig as a worker are not even considered by lawmakers in this country (yet they are in Canada or France). This is just as well, because the legal "rights" of working people in this country exist primarily in the realm of illusion. If we lab rats were to be taken under the regular labor laws and tried using traditional organizing methods, we'd end up with fewer freedoms, making less money, and we'd be lied to by the scientists more often. But this will never happen, since the drug manufacturers dictate the laws, while the government, at this late hour in the decay of scientific ethics, just barely pretends to tell them what to do. If it served the interests of "Big Pharma" to carefully track and regularize relations with their medical meat-puppets, it would have been legislated fifty years ago. On the other hand, it takes the human research subject to a higher level of civilization when he or she looks in the mirror and sees the face of a specialized worker, whose craft has its own wondrous history, its own jargon, and its own weird little culture.

Without the involvement of human subjects (healthy or sick, living or dead) modern medical science simply would not exist. We have as much reason to take pride in our contribution as do any other players in the healing professions. The purpose of my journal has been to illuminate this fact in the minds of my fellow guinea pigs.

I was stunned at the overwhelmingly positive reception reviewers, publishers, and various professionals gave to *GPZ*. I must confess that I've not made the best use of all this attention, and it's been quite a lot of attention in comparison with what I had reason to expect (you'll see as you read through this anthology). I believe that the journal has succeeded because it has an inherently interesting focus, because I have put a great deal of time and energy into each issue, and because people will generally communicate at the best level they're capable of when they can write whatever they please. It's the power of the zine. I based my journal on earlier zine models, namely *Dishwasher* and *Temp Slave!*, both of which treated unglamorous jobs as the platforms of culture. These are jobzines, and when they are done well, they empower the toiler in a unique way.

I've had a few very enjoyable experiences as results of this publishing project. One such adventure was getting sued by a fat cat in the medicine business just before his empire collapsed. Another was getting calls from hundreds of reporters, science professionals, talk-show hosts and film makers who wanted to hook onto me for various reasons. *GPZ* received all this attention because I was the only one talking on a reasonably serious level about this dark little corner of modern science from the subject's own viewpoint. The zine and I have exposed some of the dirt, and perhaps more importantly, a bit of the everyday, mundane side of being a human guinea pig.

On the grand scale of things, I realize that my input has been constructive but small. The great stand has been taken by professional journalists who have shown the public that medical science is every bit as corrupt, for example, as the oil business or the aluminum siding business. In the five years since *GPZ* has been in existence, the prestige of physicians has dropped very far below the imperfect point where it was, and now only the most utterly gullible people on earth put old-fashioned trust in their doctor's advice.

As I write, I am preparing to enter a 4-week, in-house study for a cholesterol drug, and the study includes three endoscopies, a bodily invasive procedure. Indeed, guinea pigging has parallels in the sex industry. Judging by my compensation, I'm higher up than a crack-whore, lower than a porno film performer, more brave than a phone-sex lady, and a shoe-size more lazy than an exotic dancer. In any event, I'm just another piece of meat to the corporation that pays me to be penetrated.

I, of course, am a healthy control subject who gets paid to volunteer for drug research. This makes me not quite safe but far less vulnerable, and gives me many more options, than those who offer their afflicted bodies to the white-coats, or who believe that they're getting standard treatment but aren't. I bow my head to the cancer patients whose lives are deliberately shortened so that the hospital can hang onto its research grant pipeline; to the children who die in reckless vaccination experiments (and whose skin is almost always brown); to the now-famous young hero Jesse Gelsinger, killed in a gene-therapy experiment by greedy doctors and a sneering bioethics professor. This book mentions only the tip of the iceberg, a small part of the generations of human lab rats whose existence has come to our attention. No one will ever know how many people have been lied to, manipulated, poisoned, and killed by unethical medical researchers. The best we can do is to know that they lived and suffered, to remember them whenever we step across a doctor's threshold.

In closing, I would like to express my sincere gratitude to Alexis Buss for laying out most of the pages and all the covers of *Guinea Pig Zero* since the beginning; to the several generous benefactors who have chipped in financial support over the years; to Mr. G. K. Darby of Garrett

County Press for putting up with my slowness as an author and getting this anthology to happen; to an obscure local copy shop, Pinko's, for giving me all those breaks on prices for several years in their blind love for zine publishers; to Claude Guillaumaud for endless help during my research; and to Alison Lewis for her valuable advice, proofreading, moral support, and maintenance of the *GPZ* web site. I also must give special thanks to everyone who mailed in clippings, stories, and encouragement. Without all of you kind souls, there would be another long-winded guinea pig, but there would be no *Guinea Pig Zero*.

ROBERT HELMS
Philadelphia, July 2001

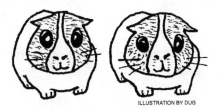

ILLUSTRATION BY DUG

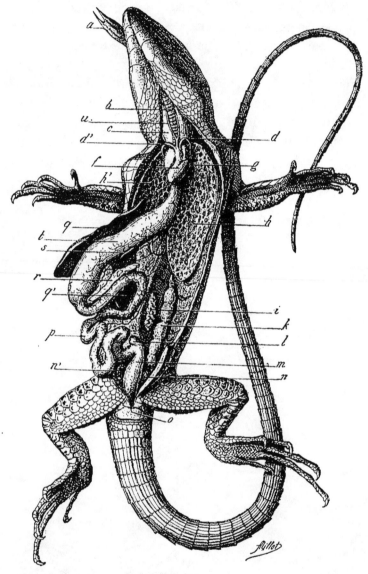

FIG. 549.

FIG. 549. — Anatomie du Lézard vert, ouvert par la face ventrale. — *a*, langue bifide; *b*, trachée; *c*, pharynx; *d*, *d'*, crosses aortiques; *g*, bronche; *f*, ventricule; *h*, *h'*, poumons; *i*, ovaire; *k*, oviducte; *l*, cæcum; *m*, rectum; *n*, *n'*, reins (petits dans cette espèce) ; *o*, écaille cloacale; un peu plus bas, la fente cloacale transversale; *p*, intestin grêle, avec le mésentère; *q'*, *q*, foie; *r*, pancréas; *s*, rate; *t*, estomac; *u*, artères carotides.

BELZUNG. — Anatomie. Phil.

TABLE OF CONTENTS

THE TREADMILL OF HISTORY

1° Les Mammifères *placentaires* ou *Monodelphes* (1 utérus) ; 2° les Mammifères *implacentaires*, divisés eux-mêmes en *Didelphes* (2 utérus) et *Ornithodelphes* (utérus d'Oiseau).

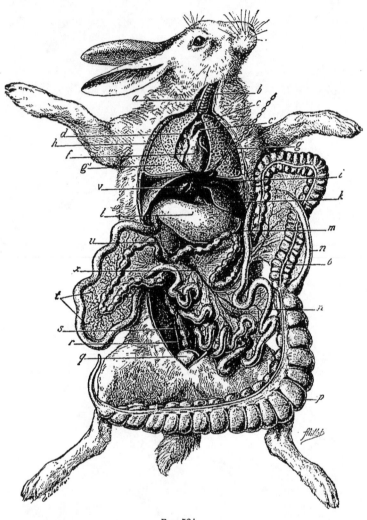

Fig. 524.

Fig. 524. — Anatomie du Lapin, ouvert par la face ventrale. — *a*, œsophage et artère carotide ; *b*, trachée ; *c*, aorte ; *c'*, artère pulmonaire ; *d*, veine cave supérieure ; *h*, section de la paroi thoracique ; *f*, ventricule droit ; *g*, *g'*, poumons ; *i*, diaphragme ; *k*, foie ; *l*, estomac ; *m*, rate ; *n*, *n*, intestin grêle ; *o*, gros intestin ; *p*, cæcum, très long ; *q*, vessie ; *r*, uretère droit ; *s*, rectum ; *t*, pancréas, rameux ; *x*, veines intestinales dans le mésentère ; *u*, rein droit ; *v*, vésicule biliaire.

RESEARCH UNIT
REPORT CARDS

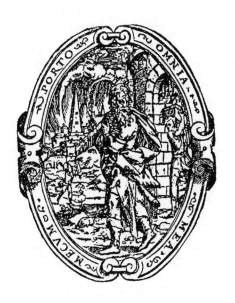

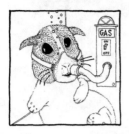

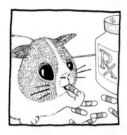

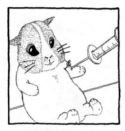

ILLUSTRATIONS BY DUG

Research Unit Report Cards:
The What, Why, and How of the GPZ Grading System
BY ROBERT HELMS

Everyone hates to have their behavior closely analyzed, except when the results are sure to be positive. If an inspector is sent into an institution by a regulatory agency, if a "mystery shopper" comes in to check up on the politeness of retail store employees, or if a postal inspector poses as a regular mailman, the parties under surveillance will get nervous, and sometimes offended. If, on the other hand, one's restaurant is written up in some arts and entertainment magazine, it's usually understood that the reporter won't be dropping in just to destroy a reputation, but is actually trying to locate good dining for the readers.

Guinea Pig Zero wishes to find a constructive balance between these two approaches. I have no interest in restricting my input to praise, since this would promote volunteering for experiments as an occupation and create more competition for myself. At the same time I would not be taken seriously if I just took cheap shots. Besides, the typical clinical research establishment is neither a sweatshop nor a war zone.

The need exists for a set of standard expectations to be set down in an independently controlled, guinea pig-based forum so we volunteers can reign in the sloppy units in a way that doesn't bring ourselves harm. Having said this, let's take a look at several units, all of which happen to be in the United States. The information offered about each unit is based on conversations with many guinea pigs; is intended to reflect the views generally held by reliable study subjects; and is not limited to my own opinions and observations. There is now an ever-growing network of

GPZ operatives. Right now one is rolling up her sleeve by the Golden Gate while another carefully inspects a protocol in the Big Apple, and still others pick up their pay in the Keystone State and then carpool it out to the Windy City. These unvanquished souls are almost everywhere, watching and remembering, giving their ears to some, but their voices to other guinea pigs.

We encourage prompt and efficient administration, ample compensation, and an atmosphere of mutual respect from the research units we frequent. A research staff's creative energy should be devoted to those ends. We discourage and condemn the following Nine No-No's:

1) Payment below $200/day
2) More than one office to deal with
3) Very bad food
4) Excessive security
5) Mediocre staff skills
6) Evasive behavior or wording related to informed consent
7) Changing the dates of a study without paying us for the hassle
8) Extra visits for procedures that should be handled during the screening day
9) Evading responsibility when something goes wrong

The report cards are based upon those criteria, and are humbly compiled by your faithful editor, GPZ*.

---

* In 1996, when this was written for issue #2, Robert Helms was still publishing the zine under the nom de plume "Guinea Pig Zero."

In Hell With a Broken Back: MCP/Hahnemann (Jointly run by Medical College of PA and Hahnemann Hospital; testing drugs for CIBA-Geigy)
BY GPZ*

FINAL GRADE: "A Big, Fat F"

This unit's problems overwhelm us in their number. Located in a psychiatric facility, one needs a visitor's pass to enter the dreary, correctional facility atmosphere of the Clinical Research Unit on the 7th floor. MCP recruiters will read off a questionnaire in a bored tone when you call, and then keep you waiting for ages when you arrive so that they can go through the explanation just once to a group of volunteers instead of dealing with each person as though they each might be distinguishable from one another.

They change the dates of a study after you've been accepted, in a nonchalant manner and without paying extra for the change. "Oh, didn't you hear about the change? It's been moved to the twenty-first. That's not a problem, is it?" Respectable units will call to tell you immediately, and throw in about $100 for the hassle.

They'll keep you waiting for half an hour for a single blood draw that you've come all the way out there to repeat. Sure, they have other things to do, but they should stop and do the 5-minute procedure so you can be on your way. Staff behaviors will either demonstrate that they value the guinea pig's time or that they don't. MCP flunks miserably in this department, too.

Sometimes they're sloppy on the venipuncture.

---

* Pseudonym for Robert Helms, Summer 1996. This piece precipitated a libel suit about one year after its original appearance. See "The Good, The Bad, and The Gutless" in this anthology.

Contacts tell us that the regular day staff might lean out with the end of the needle while using a vacu-tainer, as suddenly you hear a loud sucking sound as air instead of blood is being drawn into the tube. We know of nursing students working in research units, who would do a better job blindfolded.

There's a history of violations, like being caught taking bribes to ignore or falsify drug screen results. The entire staff was purged and replaced at least once over the past few years in order to appease the FDA and avoid closure.

The guinea pig applicant must travel to another location a few miles away to get a chest x-ray for the entry physical. On the assumption that the Medical College has a radiology department somewhere on its campus, we observe that this is an unnecessary and insulting waste of our time. We also note that most units don't require an x-ray, and we wonder why this crew always needs one. It may simply have to do with some business relationship that the unit has with another firm, or maybe the head mucky-muck has a ritualistic attachment to the procedure. In any case, a chest x-ray needlessly exposes us to that much more radiation, and at MCP it gobbles up another chunk of our day. Besides this, they always require a prostate exam! Very few research units require this unless there's a special reason connected to a study. What's a finger up the ass between friends, eh? We know they don't need to do it, but if they enjoy it, and somebody's paying for it, who cares? It's only the personal space of some ragamuffin guinea pigs.

They don't give you a copy of the protocol until you've already begun the study, and then you must ask them for it. In most units they automatically hand it over during your screening visit. They also have a strange little form where you consent to the screening routine. This is getting to be an industry standard due to certain lawsuits, but really it's the protocol of the experiment that we must consent to, not to the qualifying screen. The document used is for the whole screening process, not just for the HIV test, which has always required consent. MCP makes sure we have the bullshit sheet, but lets us pester them for the protocol. This dangerous game tries to manipulate us into thinking that a placebo document is the real McCoy.

We suggest that this hell-hole be shut down for good!

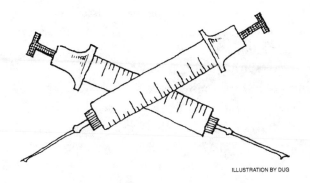

ILLUSTRATION BY DUG

La Creme de la Creme:
Thomas Jefferson University*
BY ROBERT HELMS

FINAL GRADE: "A Sparkling A"

The crew at Jefferson knows the meaning of the word "respect." If you are reliable, this is the best unit in the area. If you're unreliable, you don't deserve them.

It's a small unit of eight beds, with a separate phone line for the volunteers and usually another during late shifts (this beats a public pay phone for most purposes). In addition to what's on the house list, four videos can be rented each day from a nearby store that has a great selection. There's also a separate TV for video games. If you want some quiet, all you need to do is go to your bed and shut the door; happily, there are no TVs in the bedrooms.

Compensation is at the high-end of things, around $200 per day for inpatient time. There's a few weeks of waiting for the paycheck because, we suppose, they're part of a hospital complex and have to get their cash out of some slow machinery. The studies are usually around 6-10 days long. If they had you fasting for a while, they'll sometimes throw in a meal ticket after the discharge for the hospital's cafeteria down the block, and their food isn't bad.

Excellent professionals staff the place. The recruiter gives you a careful rundown of the experiment, makes sure that you understand and know what to expect, and she always gives you your own signed copy of the protocol as a regular part of the screening. The nurses and techs handle your blood with a calm precision that bespeaks good

---

* This report describes Jefferson's old unit, before it was moved to a somewhat larger suite in a nearby building.

training and long experience. When you call for information you get a clear and complete answer, no matter who's answering the phone.

The doctors don't require you to get every known test done, probably because they don't need them all to accomplish their study and they don't wish to invade your person any more than necessary. Everything they'll ask you to do will happen right there in the unit. There are no peripheral contacts.

Visitors are allowed in on the slower days of longer studies. You are allowed to send out for food, within a study's dietary limits. In longer studies, the staff will take you out to stretch your legs on the hospital's property. Simple allowances like these make the guinea pig feel like a person instead of like a lab rat, and this particular bunch of pigs is on a mission to use such allowances whenever they can. This humanity, above all, is what gives Jefferson the edge over all the other units we've examined.

The SmithKline Beecham Debacle of 1996
BY ROBERT HELMS, A.K.A. GUINEA PIG ZERO

Many readers of *Guinea Pig Zero* and many journalists have asked for more details on my report of a volunteer who suffered a mental breakdown from a SmithKline Beecham experiment. I had refused to share anything beyond the essentials because it is a painful affair that a lot of people wanted to close, and discussing the case could be perceived as an attack on an unfortunate fellow traveler rather than an exposure of a drug firm. I've since changed my mind: If there's any purpose to this magazine, it's to expose the dangerous practices of some pharmaceutical researchers and to warn volunteers of hazardous experiments. Furthermore, he's no longer the same person I used to care about, and is now someone who means as much to me as I do to him—very little. I recently saw him crossing a street and his strangely bloated form seemed like a ghost, walking the earth only to mock the man I once knew. This new man has no history with me.

I think mood-altering drugs should not be taken casually, nor even used except when absolutely necessary. Plenty of healthy people would disagree in regards to their own recreational options, but it's obvious that when used to excess or in certain combinations, any mood-altering substance can cause mental illness. Furthermore, new antidepressants known as "serotonin re-uptake inhibitors" (such as Prozac) are being badly over-prescribed, not unlike Valium was in the 1970's. These are, of course, widely held opinions. The experience I'll now relate only increases my cynicism toward mood-altering drugs.

In January, 1996, I returned to Philadelphia after a month overseas to discover that my closest activist associate and best friend was reacting adversely to a SmithKline

Beecham experiment at their Philadelphia research unit. The experiment involved a combination of the antidepressant Paxil and the antihistamine Seldane. This fellow was a key person in numerous projects, some involving many people and a lot of local activist money.

I knew something was wrong as soon as I stepped into my apartment. He had been watching the place and feeding my two cats while I was away. My apartment was in total disarray; things were knocked to the floor, dishes were piled up in the sink and food was spoiling on abandoned plates. The toilet hadn't been flushed, the cats' litter box was overflowing and the two animals had begun relieving themselves on a towel that lay on the bathroom floor. I was glad to see that their food and water supply had been properly seen to, but I later learned this was done by another friend who was concerned for the cats.

I met the poor soul later in the day. He was extremely manic and had been neglecting to eat, sleep or bathe. He was chattering incessantly about grand plans of high finance and revolution, and although he admitted that the drugs were having some effect, he refused to admit anything was wrong with his grasp of reality. He said things like "I'm on the barricades and I want to see who's with me and who's not." He went to see the film Twelve Monkeys about nine times, raved about it being a mystical sign of a new historical era, and claimed the film was speaking directly to him.

Everyone who knew him was deeply concerned, and when he repeatedly sent crazed communications to prominent people on behalf of our organizations, we initiated damage control like blocking his internet access and sending out disclaimers. He became very angry, and for several days went around barking orders and "forgiving" people for perceived wrongs they had done him. He never understood that people saw his actions as pure lunacy. Then there was a sort of a truce.

During the next week several of us made a concerted effort to persuade our friend to undergo observation at SmithKline. We began by calling the research unit and describing our friend's condition. The on-staff nurse knew the man well—she had spent weeks working with him as a patient. She took down all the information, called the doctors, and told us the medical staff agreed that the symptoms did merit concern. We were asked to bring him to the emergency room adjacent to the hospital's research unit where doctors could see him right away. His mother was contacted, and apprised of the situation, and she made ready to meet us at the hospital.

Our next task was to get the star of the show to walk the half-mile down to the ER and ask to be seen by the same doctors who gave him his ticket to Planet Zork. SmithKline's unit is located in the Presbyterian Hospital compound in West Philadelphia, but it isn't affiliated with the hospital. During this whole unfortunate experience, certain sympathetic friends gave up a lot of their time to stay with him at all hours so he wouldn't get into trouble on the city's streets. These same people spoke to him now, and after an hour or so got him to go into the ER. We thought we had accomplished something, but then it all went bust. Someone called a house where several of our friends lived, explained the whole situation and asked if their van could be used. These people were mostly of the opinion that our friend might be kept pumped up with thorazine or some other brain-neutralizing stuff against his best interests or even against his will. They briefly talked among themselves, then drove out to meet our friend along a street. They talked him out of seeing the doctors, assured him he could stay with them while he got himself together and that they would defend any decision he made.

He got into their van and has never, to this day, been seen by a physician about the problem. Terrible arguments ensued between the two camps, once even getting me into a shoving match with an old friend. There is good reason to be distrustful of a big industry that has an interest in concealing its dirty laundry. In this case, since he was not violent, not from a poor family and not a member of a vulnerable population, I didn't think he was in any danger of being committed.

For about three months he traveled in Britain and Laos on his savings and the money he'd earned as a "brain slut," then returned to Philly broke.* He has never discussed what happened with me or anyone I know, save for one person who had been very close to him for many years, and she doesn't share what he says. About two dozen complex and expensive long-term projects that centered around him were left to us when he flipped out yet he has never apologized to anyone. We held a meeting to assess the damage and it came to almost $10,000 worth of unavoidable debt. Now he has about two friends left. He has rented a room about a mile from where most of his former friends live and conspicuously close to the research unit where all the trouble started. He still volunteers for drug studies at SmithKline Beecham, he's putting on weight, he watches TV, cooks, and has been sighted at dance lessons. The actual symptoms lasted about four weeks. This guy, who was my best friend, is persona non grata to me now, and vice versa. It's a pity to see someone I once considered a world-class activist turn into a couch potato with a tragic case of denial.

When I realized that SmithKline Beecham was again using him after doing such damage to his life, I became

---

* I coined the phrase 'brain slut' after the debacle.

angry. I went to the unit and spoke to Donna, the Head Nurse. She flatly refused to discuss the matter in any terms, sneering, "We deal directly with our patients," whatever that's supposed to mean. She did accept a free copy of *Guinea Pig Zero* #1, however, along with my promise that I would not let the matter lie. I learned later that the brain-slut himself was in the unit while this conversation took place, and when she mentioned my visit to him, he told her I was just a nut.

Unfortunately, the man's family has decided to participate in his denial, and they alone have the power to initiate any possible lawsuit against the corporation. The man himself, even if he's faced the problem, has been disarmed by the fact that the researchers are still welcoming him back to earn more cash. The experiment that so disrupted his life paid him about $3,200. By the way, the reader should also understand that I am now no longer eligible to screen at SmithKline.

I accuse SmithKline Beecham's West Philadelphia research unit of discharging a subject prematurely—so prematurely that his mental condition led him to cause severe damage to himself during the three weeks following his release. I will endeavor to answer the following questions:

> A) How many subjects were involved in this study?

> B) How many of the volunteers experienced mental breakdowns after discharge similar to the one described in this article?

> C) What steps, if any, did SmithKline Beecham take to ensure this kind of damage would not be done to subjects in subsequent clinical trials?

D) Was the Institutional Review Board that looked over this study and later protocols for psychiatric drug experiments at SmithKline made aware of the reports of severe adverse events after the discharge of the volunteer I have described?

E) Is it possible to obtain a copy of the original protocol for this study, dating from late in 1995, for further examination? Of course the records exist, but the question remains as to whether SKB will ever discuss the matter in good faith, and whether any agency has the will to pester the corporation over an issue as small as the mental health of one volunteer. Time will tell.

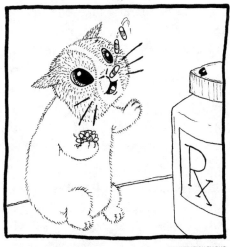

ILLUSTRATION BY DUG

Uderman's Castle: The Clinical Pharmacology Unit at Princeton, NJ˙ Controlled by Bristol-Meyers Squibb
BY ROBERT HELMS

GRADE: A Solid "A"

This unit has been around for about fifteen years and has generally maintained the same staff during that time. Some veteran guinea pigs regard the staff as close personal friends and will only volunteer at this unit. Dr. Howard Uderman, the well-liked boss, has an excellent rapport with everyone. He's so damned trustworthy and so determined to eliminate risks to the volunteers' health that you might find yourself barred from future studies because you gave too truthful an answer to a question that you would usually lie about to another doctor. Uderman, by the way, is said to be the guy who started that crazy rumor about a study where your toe is amputated and then sewn back on for $5,000. Humor being one of the qualities we value most, it may be that old Howard is the coolest doctor in the field.

The pay rate is high-end and the studies tend to be long and lucrative. The place is accessible by public transit (even if it's a bit out of the way), they pay you for the travel, and there are no unnecessary visits or procedures. There's a micro-laundromat available for free. With a TV in every 3-bed room and a layout where you can take meals in an outdoor courtyard, a long stay will not drive you mad with boredom. Another quality is it's not too big, having something like twelve or fifteen beds. There are some security rules, but nothing obsessive or disre-

---

˙The unit has since moved its facilities to another town, and its reputation has declined.

spectful. However the food is only OK.

Is there room for improvement? Not much, and certainly not in any important way. It's worth mentioning, however, that when some irregularity occurs in a guinea pig's body and the CPU sends him to the local hospital for a look, a bill will later appear in his mail slot… As if there were even the flimsiest conceivable argument for a volunteer being responsible for costs. To be fair, this has more to do with hospital bureaucracy and the predatory nature of the U.S. medical system than with this research unit. It happens not just at Princeton but all over the place. We recommend calling the billing department and teasing the shit out of them. I've never met a guinea pig who for a single moment would consider paying for a medical procedure which had any connection to a drug study.

We find this unit to be a safe, profitable, and friendly place to do our pigging.

The Anxious and the Damned
BY LISA MCELROY

Prozac has become the Valium for our age. In the 70's the middle class rose up en masse to squelch their depression with a little yellow pill. If boomers took downers in the 70's to combat stress, now they're chemically jump-starting their moods with new, overly prescribed mood-enhancers. Prozac eaters are one big lab experiment.

I decided to take the plunge into a smaller pool of subjects—guinea pigs, not baby boomers. I was curious to see how Prozac would effect my moods, and the experiment, conducted by a large metropolitan university, was intriguing: Do serotonin enhancers increase feelings of confidence in women? I was promised $100 at the end of the month-long trial. Half the group was given a placebo, the other half Prozac. Everyone met at the psych research lab three times during the trial. The meetings involved a series of exercises followed by a 3-4 page questionnaire with questions like: On a scale of 1 to 10, 1 being very unsatisfied and 10 being very satisfied, how did you feel about your performance working on the puzzle?

Usually I felt either neutral or frustrated about the whole experience. The puzzles were little blocks that had to be formed into another shape. Sometimes in the spirit of cooperation a fellow pill-gulper was called to help, and we muddled through the logic exercise, giggling at how incompetent we were. Psychological testing included writing down unusual dreams or recounting a frustrating experience and how we dealt with it. Then we gave blood (there can be no payment without some pain). But they did serve bagels and cream cheese along with some coffee and orange juice.

Besides the money and curiosity, my reason for taking

part was that women are usually not included in studies for fear of lawsuits should a subject get pregnant and give birth to some chemically altered creature. Here I thought I could do my fellow women a service. The results of this test would be women-based, with dosages based on women's body weights, women's metabolisms and women's hormonal make-ups.

Here's where the problems arose: I have a really fast metabolism. I usually feel the effects of any given drug in less than 20 minutes. It was obvious I was getting the Prozac and not the placebo. At first this pleased me, but after three days I was cursing my ill luck. I'd take a pill and 15 minutes later the back of my neck-muscles clenched, my shoulders tightened and I ground my teeth. I sweated. My mind raced. Everything had an intensity that was definitely not pleasant. It was like this time I took all-natural allergy pills chock-full of ephedrine—my sinuses cleared up, but at what price?

I couldn't sleep and I was full of the emotion we all experience in this modern world: anxiety. Only I was FULL of anxiety. Just seeing a dirty dish in the sink made me tense. This isn't worth a hundred dollars, I thought as I phoned my lab contact. No one was there, so I left a message on the machine and waited; after all, this was an experiment involving new chemicals, my brain and my overall health. I waited for three days, left another message, then got through to someone who gave me a pager number. I paged my contact and waited four more days—that's a long time to wait for a page to be returned. Meanwhile I stopped taking the pills; I didn't want to have to get extensive therapy to come off my anxiety plateau.

A weekend came and went. I called the number again and got a nice receptionist. She was full of concern, and a few hours later my contact gave me a call and apologized for the unanswered page. She explained that she had gone on vacation and gave her pager to a substitute lab contact, but the substitute inexplicably turned off the pager, hence the unanswered call. At least I knew exactly what was going on—nobody cared.

I described my symptoms and my contact hmmphed and harrumphed. "That's very unusual," she said. "I've never heard of anyone experiencing that."

"Well," I explained, "obviously I'm on Prozac and am having an adverse reaction to it."

"We don't know whether you're on it or not," she said, sly one she was. "Why don't you stop taking it and see if your symptoms go away?"

"I did," I admitted. "They did."

"Well..." she pondered, "we don't really know, so why don't you try again and see if you feel the same way."

Idiotically, I agreed. I must have really needed the money. I took another pill and 10 minutes later BOOM! I was having another anxiety attack. I paced my living room sweating. It was a terrible state, anxiety with no meaning. I looked at the phone, ground my teeth, called my contact, got the machine, and paged her again. She called back and suggested I take half the dosage. This seemed reasonable, so I cut a pill in half, which just made it crumble to dust. She recommended I mix it in orange juice. I was supposed to be taking three pills a day, but now I was down to half a pill every 24 hours. I drank my juice, which the pill made bitter, and 20 minutes later my neck was rock-hard and my stomach was in knots. My body was really rejecting this drug.

I called my contact again and told her I couldn't deal with this anymore. She agreed that maybe I was on Prozac and should quit the study, and she'd pay me $50 for the two blood tests I'd given. "Deal," I said.

"Although this is highly unusual..." she continued, "I'm going to have to ask someone about this..."

"Fine," I said, and threw the rest of my dosage away.

Two weeks later I received a phone call from an older man, a doctor working on the study. I related my reactions to him, and he matter-of-factly stated that yes, those were all symptoms that some people experience on Prozac. "Sometimes the symptoms dissipate with time," he explained. You mean my muscles clenching up into knotty ropes? The misery of just being alive? The speediness without the rush of good speed? "Muscle tension is quite common," he explained, bored with the conversation. I could tell that I was keeping him from more important duties.

"Well, it's pretty scary," I offered, in case he wanted to write it down for future reference.

"All right then, good-bye," he said.

A month later I got my check for $50.

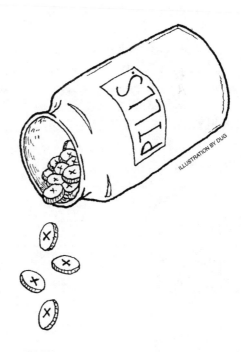

ILLUSTRATION BY DUG

Awake With A Vengeance
BY DONNO

Last Fall, while trying to figure out how I was going to scrape together the money to fly to England for my brother's wedding, I stumbled upon an ad in the *Daily Pennsylvanian* for sleep studies at the University of Pennsylvania. They needed healthy non-smokers for 3 day to 3 week studies on sleep deprivation, and I needed cash, so I made the call and made my lap around the exciting world of human guinea pigging.

An appointment was made for me to begin a rather lengthy screening process, wherein I answered battery after battery of questions concerning my sleeping habits, eating habits, recreational drug use (they actually asked If I had ever smoked catnip), my emotional states, and then they asked them all again in two or three more variations on the same questions. I was interviewed by the two principal investigators separately, and scheduled for a follow-up visit and a physical two weeks later. In the meantime I was to wear an "actigraph" on my wrist to monitor my daily cycles of activity; keep a sleep diary every night before bed and every morning after waking; and also call in to their answering machine right before bed and as soon as I woke up. In addition, I had to eliminate caffeine and any recreational drugs I might use from my life. I was being compensated for this at a rate of $2/day plus about $20 for screening days.

Shortly before my second visit, I received a call informing me that I had passed all their tests, that I appeared to be "psychologically robust," and that my blood and urine samples had come up clean—I admit I had to work hard for that clean urine! So I was in.

I ended up doing two studies for them a couple

months apart. The first was the more difficult of the two. I was confined to a hospital room in the Clinical Research Unit of the Hospital of U. of Penn, in a "time free," low light atmosphere. "Time free" means that I was completely cut off from time clues: in a dimly lit room for ten days with no clocks, TVs, radios, phone calls or natural sunlight. For most of the time during the study I had one or more of the following items attached to me: An IV with a heparin lock to facilitate hourly blood samples; electrodes on my face and head attached to a tape recorder hanging on a shoulder strap; a rectal probe (thermometer) that I got to insert myself, which then had a wire running up my arm and down my back where it plugged into my actigraph; and occasionally an oxymeter (for measuring the concentration of oxygen in my blood) clipped onto my finger. For the first three nights I was supposed to get baseline sleep of eight hours per night.

Let's review here: things taped to my face, stuck in my arm, clipped to my finger, and lodged in my rectum, in a strange bed in a strange room, and I'm supposed to sleep well? Let's just say that I did my best and enjoyed the sleep I got, knowing that when I woke up on the third day I wouldn't be allowed to sleep again for 88 hours—that's right, 88 hours, or 3 and 1/2 days. Throughout the study I had to perform tests every two hours on the computer: reflex tests, short term memory tests, psychomotor vigilance tests, tests where I just stare at a dot for 60 seconds without supporting my head with my hands, tests that are designed to be difficult or impossible to do when deprived of sleep. After the 88 hours, we got 14 hours of recovery sleep for three nights, then an 8-hour night's sleep, then we were on our way home.

The second study was similar, but much easier: 20 days, 14 of which were restricted to 4 hours of sleep each night. No rectal probe, no IV; phone calls, TV and radios were allowed; lighting was at normal levels. More importantly, I wasn't confined to my room, but could roam the CRC freely, visit with the guinea pigs in the next room, and make daily walks across campus to see the primary investigators. This helped to eliminate the cabin fever and aided greatly in remaining awake. The in-hospital phases of the studies paid about $100 per day, plus I was fed three times a day and given snacks at night during the deprivation, so I was eating a lot better than usual. I gained seven pounds during the first study, so I picked my menu more carefully the second time and gained only one.

Many people I've talked with since the study have had the same reaction: "I could never do that. I'd go crazy!" Well, if truth be told, I did go crazy—absolutely friggin' nuts. I kept extensive notes on the things going on, and upon re-reading them I was amazed by how obviously my mental capacities were crumbling. I couldn't complete thoughts. Forget about spelling and grammar, I couldn't even make sense. At one point I actually fell asleep while writing and continued writing in my sleep! From what I've been able to decipher, it looks like I wrote "...but then cows Kelly clown," though that has no obvious meaning to me. Some of my other notes included (in chronological order):

"I had another couple hallucinations today—first I thought there were spiders crawling on my computer monitor, which scared me (they were big, and not lovable like Charlotte in anyway). Then, while I was doing the math test during one of my bouts, I was staring at the screen (which is blank with white numbers flashing on it), and suddenly I felt like I was just zooming in really quickly and the screen looked like an Atari, simulating flight in open space like the whole thing was whooshing around me starting from my focal point. I didn't feel good about that one."

"I figured out what I'm gonna do if I ever have kids. Come late November I'm gonna start depriving them of sleep. By Christmas time they won't want GI Joes and Hot Wheels Cities and Tickle-Me-Elmos—no, sir. The only thing they'll fucking want is a good night's sleep."

"The last thing I ate on the outside was a corned beef special from Koch's Deli that was so good I almost cried! I had a corned beef special in here that was so bad I almost cried. Corned beef specials seem to get me all choked up these days."

"I've been hallucinating more and more recently ... while staring at the screen, my unfocused eyes suddenly focused on the reflection of my eyeball and skin inside the lenses of my glasses, and my weakened brain interpreted the image as tarantula legs coming down onto my face. Scared the shit out of me!"

"You know what's a worse edit-for-TV than Breakfast Club?—Beat Street."

"Holy moose dick, am I tired! I smashed my head on the wall when I nodded off today. That was humorous too. Sometimes I walk into doors and stuff to worry the monitors. Always fun."

"I'm zoning out and just staring at the paper. Yesterday I think I was in a trance. The monitor said it was time to fill out our sleep diaries, and I didn't respond, so she walks over to me and looks right into my eye—I'm awake and all—and starts saying, 'Don? Don? It's time to do your diaries, Don! Don!'

"And I'm aware that she's there, it's like she's a dream, speaking an imaginary language. I finally snapped out of it when she started waving her hand in front of my eyes. It was kooky."

"I'm dying here! Fucking Dying!"

"During the bout (of computer tests) I just did, I conked out, slumped over in a chair sideways, and hit my head on the wall so hard I chipped the paint (honest)! That sucked."

"I fell asleep while walking. Walked right into a wall and woke up without falling down. Impressive, huh?"

"I think today would be a good day for them to chain a live monkey to me. I'm really sleepy."

"I've been unable to speak for a large part of the morning—it was like when I got really wacky on acid and couldn't open my mouth. Also, yesterday my whole room was sparkly—you should have seen it."

And one of the strangest: "Yesterday night I had the coolest hallucination—total body/sensory experience. On one of the bouts of questions about my mental state that you rate on a 5 point scale (not at all, a little, moderately, quite a bit, extremely), you rate how much you feel certain feelings at the moment. One of them is 'carefree.' I put 'not at all' and suddenly I was Tony Randall sitting in for Johnny Carson as host of the Tonight Show, and Dick Clark was my guest. He said, 'Now Tony; I've seen you eat Carefree gum quite a bit, at least, so why don't you change that?' So I started changing my answer, and I got all the way to 'extremely' when I realized that I was just freaking out. Neat, huh?"

Luckily for me, I had a really first rate staff looking out for me. The clinical research nurses at PENN are excellent. They do their job well and as painlessly as possible. The monitors that stayed with us were mostly work study students who were given the assignment in part because of their excellent personalities and people skills, which made them a pleasure to go crazy with, and the staff from the psychology department were the best. They bent over backward to get us anything we wanted, from books and hard-to-find movies to hoagie sandwiches from my favorite deli for super bowl Sunday and a bulb of raw garlic when I felt a cold coming on. They were surprisingly supportive of my creative outlets, which included putting murals on all the dry-erase boards in the room, and creating an elaborate mobile from an IV hanger, surgical gloves, straws, plastic eating utensils, origami swans and other debris tied together with the string from herbal tea bags. My most ambitious project was fashioning a set of bagpipes out of surgical gloves, drinking straws and adhesive tape (they were a miserable failure as a musical instrument, but it was really freaky looking, so it wasn't all in vain).

The roommates I had were also the best. It wouldn't have been possible to do alone, but having someone to go through it with made the situation infinitely more livable. When it was over I was both relieved and saddened to go. That first glorious cup of coffee seemed as though the very essence of everything good that's ever been was distilled into a divine brown liquid for my personal enjoyment, and enjoy it I did. At the same time, my world had become really small really quick in there. A fellow can get used to having people wait on him hand and foot, bringing him three squares a day and idling away the hours discussing everything from philosophy to deviant sexual practices, from football to the validity of photography as an art form. Both studies included a bonus for finishing the study, and there were paid follow-up visits too. I have no reservations about participating in another study there, and in fact I've told friends to do these studies.

You'll be happy to know that I made more than enough dough to fly to my brother's wedding in the U.K. and it was lovely.

[When he wrote this story, Donno was a "starving artist" in his mid-twenties who lived and worked near the PENN campus in West Philadelphia. The study he described in detail here paid $1,466.00, including the bonus for finishing. - - GPZ]

Fifteenth Street Foibles

Recently a few guinea pigs down at 15th & Sansom were told "Don't call us—we'll call you" after one pig made and screened an in-house porno film. Sounds ridiculous, but it's true. At CDS, things can occasionally go crazy—if it's not a sex scandal, it's a fistfight—and recruiter Preston Thompson has developed a rather volatile database. The rooms at CDS are set up for sleep studies, which involves videotaping patients in their beds. One clever fellow learned that his roommate was in the habit of, well, choking his chicken, so he surreptitiously turned the camera on his roommate. After taping the poor guy whacking away, the amateur film director barged in on his learned colleagues as they watched TV and played back the tape. The staff somehow caught wind of this (possibly from the sound of twenty voices howling with laughter), and they were plenty scandalized. The well-liked but overworked Preston has since been known to bar everyone in a rowdy study from future participation.

—RH
PHILADELPHIA, 1996

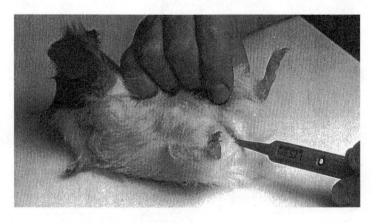

Panic At Penn
BY EMILY ELLIOT

Recently I participated in a pharmaceutical study for the University of Pennsylvania. Here in Philly the weekly newspapers are full of ads recruiting the "Tired? Depressed? Chronic Toenail Fungus?" (Honest.) I was caught by the ad for panic attacks; I've had a panic disorder for the past ten years, and it sucks. I've had to quit two jobs because of incapacitating attacks on a near-daily basis. I shake, I sweat, I can't breathe, all I can think about is running away—it's miserable. So I called up the clinic and scheduled an interview.

I went to the top floor of a nondescript building in University City, home to the University Science Center research units for Depression and Mood & Anxiety Disorder. There I met the personable director of the study, Dr. Amsterdam. He asked me a bunch of questions about my psychological and medical history and informed me no booze or Xanax would be allowed during the course of the study. "But hey, we're not always gonna be looking over your shoulder," he said with a conspiratorial wink. I like fellow boozehounds. Then he told me about the study: both the Depression and the Mood & Anxiety Disorder units were testing the efficacy of citalopram (brand-name: Celexa), a selective serotonin reuptake inhibitor (SSRI) that has been available on the market for awhile. They were researching a different molecular configuration of citalopram, the so-called "left-handed" model, which is much stronger and possibly more effective. You've heard of L-Dopa? Dr. Amsterdam told me the "L" stands for "left," but I'm not sure that's true. Anyway, this was a double-blind, three-pronged study, meaning the white powder in the huge green capsules was either citalopram, its evil twin, or a placebo, and neither I nor the doctors would know which was which.

I passed the initial interview and became Patient #001. I hung around for about an hour while various folks took my blood and urine and administered an EKG. I also answered a bunch of stupid questions about the frequency and intensity of my attacks. This was to be a ten-week study during which I was to come in either weekly or biweekly for more stupid questions. Compensation for my inconvenience consisted of free meds, or whatever was in the pills, and free "health care"—the EKG and blood draw. Big whoop. They gave me a week's worth of pills and told me to come back later.

As soon as I got home, I cracked open one of the big green pills and tasted the white stuff inside. Cornstarch. Not a trace of any bitter, chemical tang. Man, was I pissed. All that trouble for bunk drugs! Well, I figured I'd do it for a week, then go in and bitch.

The following week I went in prepared for battle. Miriam, the woman who conducted most of the weekly interviews, patiently explained to me that everyone cracks open their drugs, everyone is convinced they're taking placebos, and anyway a lot of these studies have placebo lead-ins. And on top of that, Celexa is supposed to be better than other SSRI's precisely because it does not have immediately noticeable effects. I was on Paxil for awhile, and I felt like shit for the first two weeks, so I could see her point. Okay, I thought, I'd stick it out a little longer.

By the third week I was having serious trouble sleeping. I kept waking up at like 3 a.m., then I'd be wide-awake for two or three hours. This reached the point where I could not drag my ass out of bed for school in the morning. Fortunately Dr. Amsterdam was really cool about writing notes. By this time my dosage had been increased to two horse-pills a day. Dr. A suggested I take them in the morning rather than at night, which helped this side effect eventually disappear.

Around that time I noticed another very nasty side effect: inorgasmia. In addition to a decreased libido, I was really having trouble reaching the finish line. I could eventually come, but it took forever, and sometimes I just didn't feel like bothering with the effort. I am normally fairly horny and quite orgasmic, and I had just gotten involved with a hot guy, so I was pretty upset.

Thankfully, I'm not shy, so broaching this subject with the doctors wasn't too uncomfortable. I mean, they're all professionals, but I was most comfortable talking it over with Dr. Amsterdam. He's such a dirty old man that it was fun going over the gory details. He even told me his wife had similar problems with Prozac. He had two suggestions: If the problem persisted, he could prescribe some Viagra. His other was that I should rent some pornos; he suggested that my boyfriend and I view this situation as an opportunity, a challenge that would be fun to overcome.

Quite apart from Dr. A's fatherly advice, I chose to stay with the mysterious substance in the big green capsules. This was partially because Dr. A cut my dosage back to one a day, in light of both the sleeping and the sex problems, but truth be told, I was actually experiencing less panic. By the end of the study the rate of my attacks had decreased from an average of three a week to about one in the last month. I spent less and less time worrying if I was going to freak out. I was able to eat in crowded restaurants and travel around Manhattan via the subway without taking a Xanax first. This actually means a lot to me, since my life is usually dictated by the ever-present threat of having an attack. I didn't do a 180, and I don't think I was "cured," but life has since been nicer for me, which I guess is the point.

After the end of the study, Dr. A gave me a 5-week

supply of 20-mg Celexa. I've been taking 10 mg a day. The first transition week from the study meds to the real thing definitely affected my sleep, but that was the only noticeable difference. However I am still plagued by that pesky inorgasmia thing. I often wonder if it's better to take a proactive drug like Celexa and not be able to come, or to take a reactive drug like Xanax and be a total horn-dog. The answer I've reached is yes, I'll go with the proactive, as long as the drugs are free. Once my supply runs out I'll reverse that statement. The thing is, I just don't want to have to take a drug every day of my life. With Xanax, at least it's "as needed," but the problem is that I have to wait until it's needed, at which point I'm already freaking out. I just don't know.

Overall, this experiment was a minor inconvenience. I had blood and urine taken three times over the course of three months and an EKG at the start and finish. I walked to the clinic near PENN's campus about once a week. I took a big green mystery pill every day. My main complaint is that the study was so relaxed that I often didn't know whom I'd be seeing and they often didn't know if I was even scheduled for an interview. I saw some folks only once or twice and wondered why they bothered, unless they were filling in for someone else. I wasn't informed the last day of the trial was the last day, so I went in without eating anything and was then told they needed to take blood—kind of irresponsible on their part, I thought. On the other hand, they were very flexible; I was able to have an interview over the phone while out of town, plus I felt Miriam and Dr. Amsterdam were pretty darn honest about the whole thing, accessible, and willing to answer my questions.

I am glad to see research being done in this area, but whoever wrote up the weekly barrage of questions needs to understand that these things are not entirely quantifiable.

I wish there were some room for individual response instead of rating my "avoidance behavior" on a scale from 1 to 10. I participated in this study out of a combination of curiosity and desperation. With no monetary compensation there weren't many other reasons to take part, and they wouldn't accept you if you didn't meet the chronic panic disorder criteria. The main benefit here is the free stuff, which is not trustworthy during the trial, but which Dr. Amsterdam seems happy to dole out at the end.

Spanish Fly Guinea Pig: PPD Pharmaco, Where Slackers Refuel

BY THERESA DULCE

A big operation with serious backing. Pharmaco pimps suspecting college graduates without jobs in need of money. Lots o' $ in this business. This medical research for hire thing. I've met plenty of backpack travelers who have leapt drug study to drug study across America. It's great: you get a simple physical, a place to stay, fed at least once a day, an opportunity to catch up on TV shows, and the whole time you are getting paid. The price? Surrender your freedom. You give a lot of blood. Pussies to the needle need not apply. You are operating on military time. Every comer in every room has a long, red neon clock that gives accurate time to the second. I missed a Quantum Leap rerun because I couldn't translate 5:30 p.m. into 17:30. No visitors allowed, but anyone can write you. The coordinators inspect the mail coming in, so watch the contraband. Another hazard: you are lumped in with others who need money real bad. After a few weeks (days, moments), all personalities can wear on each other. Like that non-smoking study for smokers; thirty people in-house for one month—thirty smokers who couldn't smoke, living together with only MTV to sooth them. No thanks. It was on a Sunday when I saw three different fights break out over three different college football games. I said, "Give 'em a cigarrette, god damn it!" No one would listen to me. Fine, let the boys kill each other, it's more TV for me. I liked Pharmaco. I entered in 1995, over my ass in debt. I went to Austin, grateful that there was a Pharmaco for people like me. I had my eyes on a 2-week study, and $1,500 had a nice ring to it. I got the skinny from the fat kid on the phone: Testing Ephedrine or placebo, Tolcapone, and Sinemet; fourteen days in-house; sixty blood draws in total, mostly through a catheter; $1,500.

SET-UP

In this study there are six men and six women. All twelve are sharing the same room and all are in the "big house" for the same reason—money. It's that lump check waiting for us at the end of the ride that drives us to get up at 6:30 a.m. every day to do whatever lab rats do. This gig is intense, and it's heavily staffed with phlebotomists.

At check-in we killed time till they got the urine test results. The goldenseal and the three oceans of water I'd consumed proved my urine to be marijuana-free. I didn't sweat it too much; my piss sample was so clear that I'm sure they had problems finding urine in it. The coordinators gave each of us a gray striped shirt and went through our bags—I hear that they would rather not hear that people are having sex during a study, but they won't confiscate condoms.

We shuttle from station to station every 3-10 minutes until after lunch: sit down, take pulse, check heart, get up, sit down, wait 5, draw blood, swallow pills, sit down (don't lay down), give 'em some more. The phlebs are cool. Most of them act like us when they're not in Pharmaco. Everyone moves in an orderly fashion. Each phleb is expecting one of us at an exact time. Those long, military clocks rule our actions.

The second floor of the Pharmaco building held all the in-house drug studies. It had this desperate, Flowers in the Attic feel to it. We'd look out the window and watch people do their normal, everyday errands. Stopping at red lights, working construction, eating at Burger King, having a beer. I didn't look out the window too much.

There are a lot of studies going on at the same time. Overall, the floor ratio was 10:1 male to female (the companies had more financial backing to research our male cousins). There was a slew of pool tables, big screen TVs, Nintendo games, and ever-occupied pay phones. If you were a lady pool player and you found another female who could shoot, you had an instant friend. I met Dawn at the tables. She was pretty good at pool, and later, we rigged an "ephi-study pool tournament."

Going to the cafeteria was something I lived for. On eight out of the fourteen days, we had to skip breakfast and were fed lunch after draining 90% of our blood. I've never been late for a meal. You'd cruise in with your gray stripes and watch the military seconds march by slowly. 16:04, time to eat! The food server looked bored and knows exactly what goes on your tray, and how much. Food intake is monitored—no second servings allowed. You're supposed to eat everything on the goddamned plate. Otherwise, it's not a controlled experiment. No Shit —it wasn't anyway, not with half the people in our study masking their drug intake from the doctors. Not when three of the twelve subjects were vegetarians. They were repulsed by the idea of meat, but still felt the strong attraction to the 1,500 bones. Every meal created a new challenge on how to get rid of unwanted gruel. One guy put a pork chop in his sock, walking out of the cafeteria to flush it down in little pieces. Other subjects would simply trade their chow with someone who cared. I was always downing the double burger, shifting my corn to no.5; no.8 shoved a bag of pretzels down her cleavage; no.4 put a cookie in his pocket, only to forget about it and sit on it later on. Personally, I hate milk. It grosses me out to look at and is a sure recipe for diarrhea. I always ditched my milk when the coast was clear. After the meal, the server, Mr. "I'd Rather B. Somewhere Else," would check the tray and fill out the "comments" section on the clipboard, stating what you didn't eat, and how much: "1/3 milk remained; 1/4 salad uneaten."

BARF

The drugs are hitting the boys harder than the girls. The ephedrine is not so bad. It's like a "bronchial medicine" cross-top, over the counter speed. Then they increased our dosage and things got funky. This is when the gents look to the mattresses. The guys claimed nausea more often than us. They retreated to their beds faster, too. We women figured we had more endurance because we get to tackle those monthly bouts of pain. I felt gross a few times but not enough to tell the staff or to pull a trash can over to my bedside. No.7 yacked loudly from the other room one morning. Later he was resting it off. That was when we all prayed for placebo. No.2 was feeling so bad that he hid the pills under his lounge during the dosing procedure. The coordinator even checked his mouth and he still got away with it, spitting the pills down the toilet later on. This made No.2 twice as sick after the next dosing—he couldn't fake it for the rest of the study.

HEP LOCK

I've got veins that are easy to find, but tough to penetrate. The phlebotomist called me "leather-veins." The hep lock is a blood-sucking contraption to be put into your best vein. The technicians try to hit on top of the arm, rather than the crook of the elbow or the bend of the wrist. I don't know if this is a way to save money or what, but I'd rather be stuck with a little needle a zillion times over using that appendage, a la Terminator. The hep lock is taped to you all day and all night for 2 nights at a time, and the phlebs lap into it for a draws sangre.

We were supposed to get hepped four times in total. My arms encouraged "hit or miss" hep attempts, with my veins holding a grudge for every phleb who took a stab at 'em. The plastic-sheathed metal tube would slide into the vein smoothly, but damn! no blood flow. The tube would clog and refuse to work. Now I'm holding up the assembly-line blood donation station and becoming a pain in the ass. Forget the arm! On day 12 my personal tally was 19 stabs for 7 hep lock attempts. One morning I had 2 phlebs on each arm and another guy had to come and take my pulse. The hero was a young stud who got down on his knees before me and had me dangle my arm towards the floor. Applying the hep lock upside down, Champ struck oil. Now I can go and ride the bicycle in place for 10 minutes with those little EKG thingies pasted to my body.

I volunteered for that study in the Winter of 1995. I don't know how things have changed, but over all, I'd recommend Pharmaco. Austin, TX is a cool town, the youth hostel was affordable and had no curfew, and ladies can strip for work, too. There are about seven nude and topless clubs in town, and a lot of them hire the same day you get there. Both Pharmaco and exotic dance clubs require a valid I.D. and social security number. Be at least 18 for this.

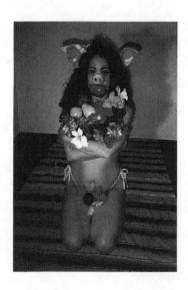

[Theresa Dulce is the editrix of Danzine, the smart & sexy journal by and for ladies in the sex business. Send $ to: Danzine, PO Box 40207, Portland, OR 97240. Web: www.danzine.org]

My Cup Runneth Over

Once in a study dosing day (I forget where), the staff was rushing to collect all of our blood samples and vital signs on schedule. They hurried from bed to bed, with no time for small talk, when something funny happened (at least I thought so): A minute or so earlier a nurse had just finished with my blood draw, and I had just thrown away my little piece of gauze. Another nurse came along to check my blood pressure, and when I suggested she go to the other side of the bed she interrupted me: "Tell me when we're not so busy, OK?" She probably assumed I wanted to tell her one of my great jokes, but that wasn't the case. The thermometer dropped under my tongue and she wrapped a blood pressure cuff around the same arm that had just given up my bodily fluids. I had tried to warn her, but it was too late. She inflated the cuff, then deep dread shaded her startled face as it was freckled bright red from the stream of blood shooting out from the fresh needle-hole. It took me a moment to think of something to say: "Not to worry, it's nice and clean. You checked it yourself, remember?" Instantly her professional composure was restored, and she calmly walked into the bathroom and washed her face.

—RH

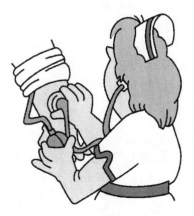

Marrow Bones
BY SAM ADAMS

Not long ago I earned a little money by donating bone marrow for research. Being generous with my bodily fluids, I had already given plasma many times and had even looked to donate semen, but it appears the unpaid volunteers have driven any paid help out of that pursuit.

Though I'll admit to a certain fascination with the procedure, my motives were purely economic. I had just moved into a new apartment after using a practice space to live in for a few months. I had lived in the practice space after sharing a place with a lovable pair of psychotics who stiffed me on my deposit. After rent and utilities, my bank account was overdrawn and I barely had bus fare to get to my temp job. The advertisement I answered said the procedure would take about 15 minutes, after which I would be paid $50. It was fairly well compensated and perfectly safe, so it seemed worth trying. After all, I'd be in the hands of the doctors at the University of Minnesota.

Like in other warm-blooded creatures, human marrow is located inside the ends of the large bones. The bulk of it is in the hips. If you put your hands behind your back and feel just above your buttocks, you can easily locate the Iliac crest, which projects outward on either side of your back and comes very close to the skin. Due to the thin tissue above the bone and the thin walls of the hips themselves, doctors have found that live marrow cells can be easily taken from a human being through a small incision just below the crest. Some people, mostly leukemia sufferers, have marrow extracted for autologous transplants. This means that their own marrow cells will be re-introduced into their body following radiation treatments and/or chemotherapy. Others donate their marrow either for love or money. For these motives, there is a different method and level of public concern.

Those giving marrow out of love are usually trying to save the life of a relative with leukemia. Donors of this type undergo general anesthesia, then bilateral incisions are made in the hips and some impressive surgical plumbing is attached to extract a few pints of marrow. The donors must then spend about a week in bed, and humane workplaces in the United States (including unionized ones) commonly grant unpaid leave to employees who donate bone marrow for a transplant. While the circumstances are stressful, the atmosphere surrounding such a donation is one of love and concern. It is a modestly heroic action, the sort of sacrifice that makes families and communities function. Then there are people like me who give marrow because they need cash. Though common enough, this gets little attention, no doubt from the state of denial surrounding most economic issues in America. I made my appointment, arrived at the emergency room (which I thought was a rather ominous place for this procedure), and filled out a form. It included a disclaimer stating I accepted all risks and would assume all medical expenses should anything go wrong. That seemed strange, but I signed anyway. I rather hopefully figured this was a common and safe procedure.

I waited in the lobby next to a coughing, sniffling guy who looked beat. I hoped the marrow extraction would not weaken his immune system to the point that he became seriously ill. We were ushered into the ER itself, where two doctors waited by empty beds. My doctor, a smiling and athletic young fellow, pulled the curtain shut and directed me to lie face-down and pull my trousers halfway down my ass. He explained the procedure while painting my hindquarters with disinfectant. I would receive several injections of lidocaine, then a tiny incision would be made just below the Iliac crest. Next a needle would be inserted through the incision and into the surface of the hipbone, and about a cup and a half of marrow would be aspirated into several syringes. The lidocaine injections would cause the most discomfort, he said, though there might be an "odd" feeling as the marrow was aspirated due to the momentary vacuum inside my hip.

He asked if I was a student, and I told him I was a medical transcriptionist. He seemed puzzled by this. "I guess this is just something you had to try once, huh?" he asked. I offered no argument. It was 7:30 in the morning, I hadn't had coffee yet, my pants were pulled down, and I didn't feel like discussing my life with this man. Doctors as a rule seem uncomfortable discussing the economic circumstances of their patients and subjects, and in this case the feeling was mutual. Since I wasn't a starving student and was actually an "office professional," he probably thought I had a decent income, health insurance, a car and a home in the suburbs like most of the clean-cut young white males he encountered. The fact I was here doing this for cash meant I was at least a rather strange person. Instead of challenging him, I just waited for him to do his job so I could pull my pants up and leave.

For a moment he stepped away and I heard voices. He returned and asked if it was all right if an intern observed the procedure. "Sure," I said, "the more the merrier." I am not terribly squeamish, and I figured he'd be less likely to fuck up with one of his colleagues watching him. The intern, an attractive young woman, introduced herself to me, and then we began.

The injections were as painful as promised. Too many desk jobs, along with my part-time musical pursuits, have begun to irritate my Sciatic nerve. Being poked with needles didn't help, and I wriggled and yelped a bit. I was too tender to proceed without a second round of lidocaine, which did the trick. The doctor then sliced into my unfeeling flesh and crunched down into my hip. "OK, we're in," he said. "Now comes the aspiration." Pulling the plunger on the syringe, he swiftly began extracting marrow. The "odd" sensation he had described was in fact exquisitely painful, causing what felt like a strong electrical charge to run up and down my hip and thigh. Back in my meat-eating days at my parents' table, I used to love cracking the ends of duck and goose bones and sucking out the sweet marrow; perhaps the birds were having their revenge on me. I crammed my face into my pillow and began to softly voice obscenities and invoke Deity.

"Are you all right?" asked the doctor. I wanted to say, No, there's a needle in my hip; let's finish and remove it, please. Instead I said, "Yeah, I'm just not digging it." "We're almost done," he said in the loud teacher's voice that indicated he was addressing me and not the intern. He had been chatting brightly with the intern, and I wondered if after they were done with me they'd have brunch and talk of children and recreational vehicles.

Finally, he removed the needle and taped gauze over the incision. "Glad you could join us today," I mumbled to the intern, who smiled and left. As I gingerly sat up and put on my glasses, the doctor explained the study in greater detail. The researchers were studying the marrow cells that produce leukocytes. Eventually they might be able to control production of these cells, which would result in better treatments for a number of diseases. I suspected that I and most people I know would never benefit from this research, but certain drug firms and insurance companies might benefit greatly; I just smiled and said I was glad to do my part for humanity. I took a good look at the syringes full of my marrow, but was fairly unimpressed; marrow looks just like thick blood.

"Okay, sign here," he said. "Your check will be out in

about two weeks, once accounting approves it." My jaw dropped. Somehow, I had assumed that "after the procedure" meant I would be paid immediately upon completion. Always, always read the fine print.

I signed the form and walked out into the sunshine, where I treated myself to a cappuccino before catching the bus to work. "You'll feel like you've been kicked by a horse," the doctor had warned me, and I sat very stiffly and carefully for the rest of the day.

Certain experiences seem to teach me nothing except not to repeat them. I had done little for my immediate financial troubles and had made the morning quite unpleasant. Since that time I've had no ill effects, but I have avoided donating this or any other bodily fluid, and have resolved to never in my life crack a marrowbone again.

Abbott Laboratories

BY DISHWASHER PETE (VETERAN OF A 16-DAY STUDY)

FINAL *GPZ* GRADE: "Pretty Decent"

LOCATION:

Forty miles north of Chicago and not far from Abbott's massive drug manufacturing plant, Abbott's research unit is located within the Victory Memorial Hospital in Waukegan, Illinois. (When I called my mom and told her where I was, she said, "Waukegan? That's where Jack Benny's from!") The hospital is about a mile north of the commuter rail station. A one-way trip from Chicago runs about $5. There's a Greyhound stop on the far side of town. It took me about two hours to walk from there to the hospital but I was walking pretty slow so as to not get my bilirubins too excited for my screening.

FACILITY:

Encompassing the entire north wing of the hospital's third floor, the facility can be accommodating when it isn't filled to its 60-odd capacity. The day-room, pool room, dining area, and (unfortunately) reading room have TV's and VCR's. The staff rents five suggested videos a day from the local Blockbuster. The best place for peace and quiet away from the TV's is out in the waiting area. Visitors are allowed during the day. There is one (Bell) pay phone and one regular phone available.

PAY:

The study I did paid $2,500 for a 16-day stay, which came to $150 a day. There was just one quick outpatient return two days later. They sometimes pay better and they also have studies that are nothing but outpatient visits, though I'm not sure how well they pay for those. Abbott pays $25 for a screening regardless of whether or not you make it into a study.

RECRUITMENT:

Abbott has a toll-free telephone number but it's often difficult to get anyone on the line. I suspect that when they don't have any studies going on, they simply don't answer the phone. The screening process is routine. After I screened, I left town. When I was accepted as an alternate, I worried I might travel a thousand miles back only to not be accepted into the study. I gambled, though, and eventually made it in. Word about Abbott's studies apparently gets around, since there were guinea pigs from New Jersey, Pennsylvania, Indiana, Maryland, Kansas, Wisconsin, and even one guy that had come all the way up from Miami.

CONSENT:

The consent was done in a respectable one-on-one fashion. After the study got under way, the unit's head doctor and a guy from Abbott's research division lead a discussion on exactly what the study was all about. Initially I expected the meeting to be heavy on mumbo-jumbo and evasive answers. Instead, what transpired was an extremely interesting discussion. The doctor and the researcher did their best to explain themselves as thoroughly as possible in easily understandable terms. The meeting went on for much longer than originally anticipated and I learned quite a lot. The questions put forth by my fellow pill-poppers were so intelligent and so thoughtful, it made me proud to be a guinea pig.

SECURITY:

After the initial bag search during admissions, there is no overbearing show of security. There are no security goons or cameras or anything like that. About the only notable security measure is that the front door is locked at night. Not wanting to be baby sitters, the Abbott staff expects responsible behavior from the guinea pigs. As a result, there is a high degree of mutual respect between the staff and the guinea pigs.

SKILLS:

Top notch. All of the staff were extremely skillful, courteous, and knowledgeable. In fact, unlike the staff at certain other units I've been to, they never once grumbled while trying to attach the EKG electrodes to my hairy chest. (The trick is to mat down the hair with rubbing alcohol just prior to attaching the electrodes.)

ATTITUDE:

The only downside was the head nurse and her bad attitude. She needlessly stirred up trouble several times. I meant to write a letter to Abbott complaining about her but I've since forgotten her name. Otherwise, the rest of the staff was great.

FOOD:

Generally, the food was good. But on that very first day, when I wasn't sure exactly how strict they were about their clean-plate policy, I ate the most horrid concoction ever— some sort of soupy coleslaw. And it wasn't just me. Even coleslaw lovers complained. Although there was always a staff member watching us during mealtimes and checking our trays to make sure we'd eaten everything, it was pretty easy to dump the coleslaw during its subsequent appearances. But like I said, for the most part, the food was good.

SUMMARY:

Overall, I had a pretty good experience. The best part was on Wednesday afternoons when elderly volunteers conducted bingo games in a studio in the hospital's basement that were televised throughout the hospital. Winners phoned down to the studio. While someone sprinted to confirm the winning card, the host read jokes from The Reader's Digest. Combs and toe nail clippers were awarded as prizes. One time a woman up on the fourth floor won three straight games, leading to a guinea pig chant of "Fixed! Fixed! Fixed!"

What They Think of Us: Sarah Wallace Interview
BY HOBBIN A. SMITH

There is a reason why we as subjects rarely come into contact with our principle investigators: That lack of contact is supposed to maximize the objectivity of the data's analysis. On March 11 The Seattle Times printed a story about some apparently unethical practices at the Fred Hutchinson Cancer Research Center that lead to the deaths of some test subjects. In December I interviewed a study coordinator from the Hutch, Sarah Wallace. At the time she expressed surprise that anyone would think Hutch employees would not respect their subjects. I still believe that Hutch employees have nothing but respect and concern for their subjects, but that desire for objectivity could be the source of such tragedies. Objectivity can help keep data from being muddled, but hardened objectivity also leaves everyone involved outside of the experience and unaware of any problems in a protocol. When questionable practices are taking place, it may be that the coordinators and nurses we work with are just as ignorant of these problems as we are.

I attempted to reach Sarah Wallace to see if she could add anything to her previous interview, but she was in the hospital having a baby and was unavailable for comment. The following is the text of the December interview with Sarah Wallace, Research Coordinator of the Pain Research Laboratory at the Fred Hutchinson Cancer Research Center:

Hobbin: What do subjects do that you really appreciate?

Sarah: What I really like is when somebody goes above

and beyond. When they really pay attention to what you are doing and take it seriously. Like, they aren't just doing what they have to for the money, but also recognize that they are participating in research and that the data is important, so they'll really put a lot of thought into their responses. Then later, when we're looking at data to see what to use again or to help design the next study, we can look at that person's data and say "okay, I know this data is really good," so we can base our decisions on what they say. I also really like it when we have Hutch employees because they understand that it's data, so they are very careful with their responses. That's the dream subject.

Hobbin: Don't we all strive to be the dream subject?

Sarah: The answer to that question is a definite "no."

Hobbin: What do subjects do that you really hate?

Sarah: Definitely "no shows" are the most irritating. And because our days are so long, when they show up like an hour late. Also, extremely irritating subjects; you're stuck with this person all day, you try to make it a pleasant experience for them, but it's really hard when you have nothing in common. Like there was this one guy in particular. His personality was irritating and it just didn't get any better. He was just so weird! There was a just lot of stuff about him that was strange. But that's pretty rare.

Hobbin: What is your opinion of subjects in general?

Sarah: I really enjoy the subjects—that's my favorite part of the job. I get to sit and talk to people that I don't usually talk to in a normal setting. Like we've just had a bunch of artists; it's not stuff I get to talk about in any other setting. There's one musician that is really into vegetables. He knows all these interesting facts about different vegetables. He has a web page where he does a vegetable of the week. There was also a performance artist, which is something I completely don't get, so this person was explaining what it's all about. It was really interesting. I definitely enjoy the vast majority of subjects.

At the end of our interview Sarah asked, "So what's the deal? You get one issue of *Guinea Pig Zero* and suddenly you're writing for it?" I explained there is a lot of press about researchers that have mistreated and disrespected their subjects; I wanted to do an article or two about the researchers, investigators, coordinators and nurses that do respect their subjects. Because she has the highest respect for her subjects, Sarah was shocked to hear about investigators and staff that have no regard for what their subjects go through. She was also shocked to learn that subjects may assume the Hutch research staff would be similarly disrespectful because of horror stories they'd read in the press.

"I mean, like there was one study where everybody in the lab was taking Paxil," she said. "So we're like 'Hey, this medication does x, y and z.' At the Hutch we've all done studies. That's just really funny that people would think we don't care about them or respect them.

"I guess I've been in the research world too long. It is incredibly difficult to get federal funding for these projects. Incredibly brilliant people with fantastic ideas have a difficult time getting their first grant. It's a classic Catch-22: you can't get funding because you've never had funding before. You really have to have a stellar reputation in your field in order to run your own grants. I just sort of assumed everyone would be aware of this.

"The other funny thing is we have to go through this

review process every year with the Hutch and our federal funding agencies. They review the safety precautions we have in place for our subjects and whether or not they are treated ethically."

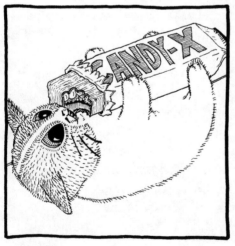

ILLUSTRATION BY DUG

The Good, the Bad, and the Gutless:
Four Months on the Barricades for a Free Press
BY ROBERT HELMS, A/K/A GUINEA PIG ZERO

Late in the spring of 1997 I was pleased to learn that *Harper's Magazine* had decided to reprint three of my "research unit report cards." The material was to be shortened from its intended length, but was given the green light for the June '97 issue. I expressed my sincere gratitude and watched for the magazine to appear on the newsstands. I've rarely read *Harper's* over the years, but knew it to be a fine and prestigious literary magazine with a pretty large circulation. My career as a writer is still in its infancy, so there was no mistaking that this was a lucky break. The biggest exposure before this had been good reviews and friendly mentions in articles about human experimentation.

Before I was able to even see the passages printed in that venerable journal, I got a real surprise in a message from one of their senior editors. Allegheny University for the Health Sciences, one of the subjects of a flunking report card, was threatening to sue *Harper's* for libel if they didn't pull the newsstand copies and apologize for what I had written. "Please call me!" he wrote. On my message index were also posts from *The Associated Press, The Washington Post,* and *The Philadelphia Inquirer.*

If I was already blushing from the exposure in *Harper's,* you can bet that getting interview requests from two major newspapers and the international news wire really had me up. I started the phone tag and jumped into the debate. At this time I had just returned to Philadelphia from France. I was sort of couch surfing at the homes of friends with my belongings stashed in about

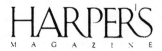

HARPER'S
MAGAZINE

December 16, 1996

Guinea Pig Zero
4728 Spruce St., #369
Philadelphia, Pa. 19139

Dear GPZ:

I'm an editor on the Readings section of *Harper's Magazine*. Readings is a sort
of cultural digest composed of everything from reprints from 'zines and
literary journals to excerpts from upcoming books to political documents.

We came across a copy of issue number 2 of *Guinea Pig Zero*; congratulations on
putting together a valuable and enjoyable 'zine. We particularly liked the
"Research Unit Report Cards," and would like to consider reprinting excerpts
from three in an upcoming issue: Medical College of Pennsylvania/Hahnemann,
SmithKline-Beecham, and Robert Wood Johnson. Of course, we would credit
GPZ.

I would love to talk to you about this and perhaps find a way to fax you a
galley copy of the excerpt we would like to run. Please feel free to contact me
either by phone, 212/614-6523, or by e-mail, susan@harpers.org.

Thanks very much. I'll look forward to hearing from you soon.

Best,

Susan Burton
Editorial Assistant

four locations, and I was out of pocket to the point of vulgarity, so getting messages quickly was not always a sure thing. I am not employable in the usual sense, at least in Philly. The number of research units (in this area) where I'm still welcome is limited, and it's never easy to just pop back into town and start earning a living again. The way I must have come off to professional journalists (and more importantly to the top executives of *Harper's Magazine*) must have been pretty down-and-out, living from one check to another, always close to the bone—perfectly in accordance with the public image of a professional guinea pig.

The day after the news of the lawsuit broke, I called collect from a pay phone downtown and spoke to two *Harper's* VP's and publisher Rick MacArthur on a speakerphone. They asked me many questions about my experiences at Allegheny/MCP. They spoke assuringly about my right as a consumer to independently evaluate a research facility, and they said although they chose the report cards for their uniqueness as literature, they were in sympathy with my cause of helping research subjects protect themselves from ill treatment. We agreed that not all of my interests were identical with those of *Harper's*, but we had a common interest in defending against censorship by some billionaire medical investor with a formidable attorney. MacArthur assured me that I was "way ahead of them," meaning we had no problems in fending off the corporate bullies. Later I would wonder why he said this.

Rick MacArthur is the grandson of the billionaire philanthropists who provided the seed money for their eponymous John D. and Katherine T. MacArthur Foundation. This is one of the ten largest charitable trusts in the United States. It regularly gives major funding to National Public Radio and other non-profits both large and small, and it dumps "genius awards" of $300,000 or so in the laps of winning minds every year, all in the course of its philanthropic business.

I am the grandson of two poor Irish immigrants and two kindly blue-collar Mayflower descendants. I'm a working stiff in the family tradition, and the reason I'm telling you this is not to say that Rick MacArthur is an evil man, but merely to demonstrate that his thoughts are not at all like my thoughts. From his perspective, I am a passing curiosity whose bio-slutting is the adventure of another class. To me, he is someone who has had, since birth, all of the advantages this civilization can provide. We can understand each other's lives only on an intellectual level. The real fabric is left to speculation.

Sherif Abdelhak, the CEO for Allegheny University (which owns about 2 dozen hospitals in Pennsylvania) paid himself $1.2 million in 1995. I've been told he is a member of the Kuwaiti Royal family and is an actual sheik, but I found out later that he isn't. There were hospital mergers in Philadelphia this year motivated only by the wish to avoid being sucked up into Abdelhak's financial empire. I also know that Allegheny is a "tax exempt, non-profit" organization, and I have a hard time reconciling a $1.2 million salary with the term "non-profit." I feel comfortable stating that he's not in the medical business for altruistic purposes.

When this oily businessman's outfit decided to sue me, they were already too late. I had published the report cards a year earlier, at which time the *Philadelphia City Paper* had run a story on the reports and the on-line magazine *Hotwired* reprinted them in their entirety. They were responding to the larger damage done by *Harper's* quarter-million readership, to the fact that *Harper's* had deep pockets, and especially to the way that *Harper's* edited my writing. The shorter version gave the reader the impression that Allegheny had broken laws regarding informed consent, but I'd never written any such thing. A press release from *Harper's* VP for Public Relations Sean McLaughlin made this worse by exaggerating the impression. These people simply had no knowledge of the human research industry, but were playing the story for what they could.

Representing the hospital was Richard Sprague; having won the largest libel award in U.S. history on his own behalf, he is really feared in media circles. He got 24 million bucks from *The Philadelphia Inquirer* because they wrote that he squashed a murder charge as a favor to a friend while second in command at the DA's office in the early 1970's. He generally protects Republican political figures and large institutions from the media. This means that when *Harper's* got a letter from him threatening to sue, they were under more than the usual pressure.

Representing *Harper's* was another prestigious lawyer, Victor Kovner. His firm handles legal matters for many New York City magazines, and he's as well connected in Democratic circles as Sprague is in Republican. With libel cases, I'm told Kovner doesn't fight it out in court, but generally 'makes the lawsuits go away.' Later I learned why he found this preferable for *Harper's* rather than standing up for them on principle alone.

The first thing *Harper's* did was release a 'clarification and apology' for the first time in its 147-year history. I was not sent a copy, but a reporter from *The Chronicle of Higher Education* read it to me over the phone. I did not feel that it meant the fight was over, and I still felt that *Harper's* was defending my rights to criticize the research units. Now I know that I was wrong about that.

For weeks after the initial conversation with Rick MacArthur, I communicated over email with a *Harper's* editorial intern, and was frequently on the phone with their spokesperson and Victor Kovner. I was consulted on details of my residence since starting the zine and on the publicity I'd received since running the report cards, and all the time I believed that we were preparing a case against the libel charges. If I were not a resident of Pennsylvania, I'd be able to have the case moved to Federal Court. This would be better for *Harper's* since PA is less friendly towards the media than most states, perhaps the least friendly. Anyway, Kovner eventually told me that it was almost finished and that he wanted to reach a settlement that included a release for me. For about three weeks this is what I was told; in the meantime, a first apology was printed in the August issue, and it was then that I fully realized how I was being trashed in this bargain. There was a build-up of displeasure in my head, and in the third week of August I made a press release stating that if *Harper's* settled, it was on their behalf, not mine, and I did not wish to be released from the lawsuit. I'm very glad I did that, because a few days later the phone rang and a reporter from *New York Magazine* asked me what I thought of *Harper's* next apology in the September issue that trashed my report card on SmithKline Beecham.

From that point on, because of their disgusting spectacle of cowardice at my expense, I have detested the editors at *Harper's*. They caved on a letter from SKB without ever discussing the text of the report card with me. *Harper's* apologies gave the impression that *Guinea Pig Zero* is some half-assed little thing that embarrassed their noble institution by passing false information in its pages. They did not apologize for their own stupidity, and they never dug any further to find out who was full of shit and who was telling the truth. This is when *Philadelphia Magazine* reporter Steven Fried got involved, to find out where the truth lay, and he investigated the story for the October issue. In a nutshell, Fried discovered that except for small errors of fact (the amount paid for the SKB study and the involvement of the FDA at Allegheny), I had hard evidence that supported every damned thing I said. He even interviewed a veteran guinea pig who said he'd personally bribed Allegheny/MCP staffers to ignore urine drug-screen results. Fried stayed on the fence with the SmithKline affair, but his article amply illustrated that my zine is exactly what it claims to be, and that *Harper's* VP Sean McLaughlin and his editorial staff caved to the lawsuit without following up.

In early September, *Harper's* settled with the hospital chain under secret terms, but certainly terms that included a large transfer of cash from the magazine to the people they feared. Allegheny is said to be "extremely pleased" with the deal. I was still being sued and got a hearing date from the court, so I scrambled to line up legal council. I found an attorney of very high repute, Sam Klein, to represent me on principle, even if I was unable to pay him, and he advised me that *Harper's* needed my consent to be cut out of the suit without me. Victor Kovner had forgotten to tell me this while pretending to act in my interests, just as he'd omitted mention of other essential details, like the letter from SmithKline Beecham. Actually, I went through the whole adventure without ever seeing the full complaint, or even knowing that I had a right to see it; I had only seen the summons. All I knew was that I was sticking to my guns, and that if it kept going it might have turned into another McLibel suit, or one that backfires on the plaintiff after trying to suppress public criticism by dragging an under-funded defendant into the legal system. Suits filed with this intent are known as Strategic Lawsuits Against Public Participation, or 'SLAPP suits.' Usually it's safer and easier to cave in than to defend oneself against such an action.

As it turned out, Allegheny waited until after the feature article appeared in *Philadelphia Magazine*, then dropped the lawsuit the day before the first court appearance in early October. They knew that there was nothing to gain from me but bad publicity, and since they were about to lay off 1,200 hospital workers they had enough of that on the way. It was the perfect time to get me out of their lives.

Looking back on the whole Allegheny affair, I have learned some important lessons and scored a few victories. One should never speak to anyone except as an equal. I knew that already, but I let the rule slide when dealing with *Harper's* and their attorney. On the brighter side, the lawsuit has generated an enormous amount of good publicity for my zine, but I should note that there already was a good deal of exposure before the suit began. I don't owe the zine's success to Abdelhak and MacArthur, but they have turned up its publicity volume a bit. Reporters (and lately the entertainment industry) are continuously contacting me. I have no idea if I'll be able to turn this into a steady income, but it certainly seems like a possibility.

The effectiveness of the report cards has been proven beyond a doubt. I was actually inclined to stop doing the cards, thinking that they had made the point and continuing would be redundant. Then they hit the national media. Just last week I was interviewed for a cover story in the *Pittsburgh City Paper* (Nov. 20-27 1997 issue), and I read the most eloquent compliment I've ever received when my complimentary copy arrived. I was quoted extensively, and the report card lawsuit was mentioned:

> ...the incident continues to reverberate in the research community. University of Pittsburgh Medical Center spokesperson Amy Kemp, in telling City Paper that she couldn't locate a researcher who was willing to be interviewed for this article, partly blamed 'the zine,' saying, 'It's been difficult getting

someone to speak.'

—Bill O'Driscoll, in "I was a Human Guinea Pig."

Take this to heart, fellow zinesters (especially jobzine writers)! Work hard, stand your ground, and box 'em to the ropes. It brings us together in a mutual cause, and it's an awful lot of fun.

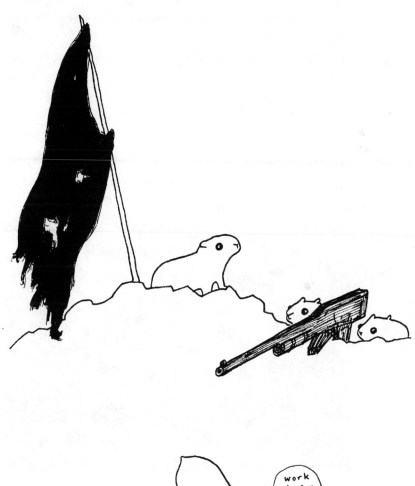

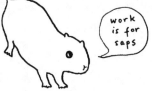

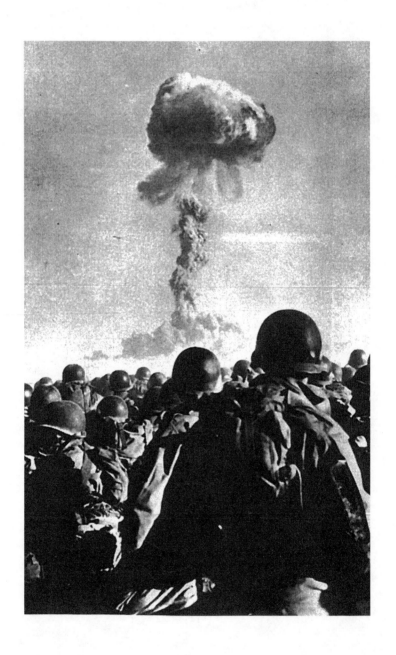

THE TREADMILL OF HISTORY

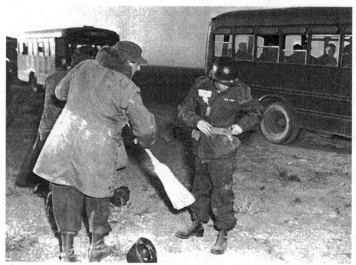

Decontamination, army style: brushing away radiation with a broom

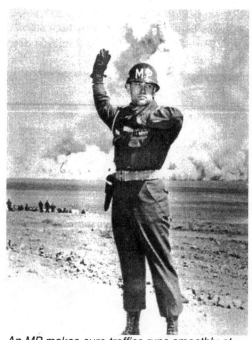

An MP makes sure traffics runs smoothly at test site.

Experimentation: Reality and the Lie
BY ROBERT HELMS

A degree of power exists at which the most infamous man finds himself protected by his own infamy.
—*Octave Mirbeau*

While passing time in a drug study in Delaware, one of my fellow volunteers spoke of his military service in various government actions and during the Vietnam War. He had been in Special Services, which means that he would often be assigned to utterly ruthless and immoral missions to which the government could never admit. He might be handed a list of names or villages and sent into a "neutral" zone such as Laos or Cambodia, where he might assassinate politically meaningful people and maybe even slaughter their families. In other words, he was a problem solver. I asked him the old familiar question: "Why did you join that particular corps—didn't it bother you?" He explained that the only way he felt that he could have even the smallest influence in the events taking place around him was either to stay entirely out of the war and desert, or to be as well-informed and personally dangerous as possible. Every day the regular enlisted men were being sent to their deaths for no reason and with no idea of what was going on in the minds of their commanders, much less in other parts of the conflict zone. He chose to be a conscious, deadly agent instead of a plate of dog food. He didn't think of it as choosing to be a homicidal maniac.

This fellow traveler's choices were none I would be proud of, and his reasoning does not excuse the atrocities he committed, but if the choice is between regular military duty or the status of an inner-circle operative, his choice has an obvious logic. Looking into certain chapters of military history, I can agree that in hindsight, any war can appear to be an absurd orgy of mass murder where only a few partisans really understand what is happening. Yet the pointlessness of death becomes more vivid whenever one hears the word *experiment* in relation to a government or institutional action.

This conjunction of military man-turned-medical guinea pig leads us into this chapter. Throughout history governments have used theaters of war and theaters of medicine as laboratories for learning new ways to deal with people, employing strategies under particular circumstances, and for testing new technology. In war, soldiers and civilians have served as guinea pigs while generals labored to reach the next threshold in state-of-the-art mass destruction. In medicine, ordinary people have served to further the knowledge of ever-searching physicians. In this story we'll examine two war experiments, one real and one *hubris* covered up as an experiment, and a medical blunder that was excused by bureaucrats as a research experiment. The reader may notice that a high level of suspicion is appropriate while reading the apologies.

We'll first look at an actual military experiment, the April 26, 1937 Nazi Luftwaffe bombardment of the Basque town of Guernica in Spain. In this instance the town's population and architecture served as the experimental matter and learning curve for the Nazi war machine. The motive for the raid was quickly surmised by outside observers, but Hitler and his Spanish client would not admit to its experimental value.

After that is the August 19, 1942 Allied Forces raid on Dieppe, France. This unauthorized mission turned into one of the worst blunders of WWII, but has been historically recognized as an experiment where key insights were learned that aided in the successful Normandy invasion two years later. In reality nothing was proven but the stupidity of the mission's commander, Louis Mountbatten (1900-1979). The raid was not an experiment.

Finally we'll see how the Dieppe raid is similar to the tragic death of Nicole Wan in 1996. Like the Dieppe case, Nicole's demise was the result of incompetence whitewashed as an experiment. Her overdose of lidocaine during a routine bronchoscopy had nothing to do with experimentation, but the 'quest for the unknown' was invoked as bureaucrats fumbled for a plausible excuse for this young woman's death. Experimentation may exonerate but does not justify ineptitude.

Guernica, the Experiment that Really Was

We live under the laws of war. It consists of massacring as many men as you can in the least possible time.
—Octave Mirbeau

On April 26, 1937, at the height of the Spanish Civil War, Hitler's air force used the Basque town of Guernica and its 9,000 civilians for military research. Guernica was the first town in history to be terrorized and destroyed by means of aerial strafing and bombardment. Located about 13 miles East of Bilbao, Guernica is a place of deep mystical importance for the Basque people; it is the spiritual capital of their race and the home of the sacred oak tree of Guernica, a symbol of Basque independence. On the day in question Guernica still lay just 6 miles within the Republican zone, parts of which were held by anarchist militias and the government of Spain, and was attacked by the insurgent right wing forces led by General Francisco Franco.

Hitler's Condor Legion, under the command of Lt.

Colonel Wolfram Von Richthofen (cousin of the famous flying ace "Red Baron" Von Richthofen), had been sent to assist Franco the previous summer, just after the conflict started. It was this Condor Legion that bombed Guernica. Unlike previous air raids that generally hit targets of military importance, Guernica's two gun factories and its bridge were among the few structures left standing by the bombs.

The raid began near 4:30 p.m. and ended near 7:30. It was a Monday, the weekly market day, so many people were outside. Bilbao had been bombed the previous day, and Guernica's main square was filled with that town's refugees waiting near the train station to get farther away from the front lines. The first bombs fell in this main square. The planes divided their tasks into three parts:

First, 23 large Junkers-52's made high passes, dropping 1,000 pound explosive bombs that blasted out the concrete structures of the buildings. Second, another squadron of experimental Heinkel-111's returned with 9-pound incendiary bombs and 2-pound aluminum tubes containing thermite and white phosphorous to ignite the wreckage of the buildings. Third, much smaller Heinkel-51 and Messerschmitt BF-109 fighter planes flew low over the town and the outgoing roads with orders to shoot "anything that moves." The fighters dropped very small anti-personnel bombs that filled the air with razor-sharp metal splinters and used wing-mounted machine guns to shoot pedestrians. During the raid panicked men, women and children were moving along the roads and through the surrounding fields; all were attacked, including livestock and the nuns from the hospital. In all, 889 were wounded and 1,654 people died in the attack. The town had no anti-aircraft flack guns and the Republican forces had only 8 planes to offer a spirited but futile resistance. The townspeople were also unaware of enemy spies, including the most influential man in the town, a gun factory owner named Rufino Unceta. Unceta kept his sympathies (with the attackers) hidden and delayed the removal of his machinery to safer ground. This way the insurgent forces could capture his fully fitted weapons plant a few days after the bombardment and add it to their already fortified arsenal.

Decades later German pilots claimed the Renteria Bridge was Guernica's principal military target. The bridge is a small stone structure held up by two small pillars, and it supposedly survived because the wind had blown their bombs off target. The question remains as to why anti-personnel and incendiary bombs would be used to destroy such a target. In fact, the mission's commander knew that the town was just 300 yards from the bridge. The small incendiaries were certain to scatter like leaves and land all over the area when dropped from 6,000 feet. Clearly, the bridge was never the real target—the town was marked for annihilation.

Von Richthofen had four Stuka dive-bombers capable of carrying single 1,000-pound bombs available to him that day, and these could have been precisely deployed to destroy the bridge. Furthermore, if the Junkers had been attacking a single, small target, they would have flown single file and not abreast as they did. Consistent eyewitness reports quickly appeared in London and New York stating whose airplanes attacked Guernica and how. The fascists denied the attack, claiming "Red incendiary" land mines and the fires caused the craters, but these denials always miserably conflicted with one another. The news caused a major stir in Catholic circles throughout the world; the Basque region is one of legendary, faithful devotion, and many clergymen who were fiercely loyal to Franco had their credibility brought into question. It must be stressed that the Spanish Nationalists and the Nazis would never disclose the actual motives for this raid any more than Hitler would advertise the Dachau death camp. The absolute amorality of the experiment is obvious.

While assisting the takeover being waged by his Spanish client Franco (who later became a U.S. ally), the Luftwaffe used Guernica to try a new "strategic bombing" system that would prove extremely useful during WWII. Important lessons regarding aircraft design and urban terrorism were also learned in this Nazi-backed experiment. Guernica became a military success, and the techniques devised there have since become basics of modern warfare used by every world military power.

Dieppe, 1942: The Experiment that Never Was

Dulce et decorum est pro patria mori. (It is sweet and fitting to die for one's country).

—*Horace*

There is something more mysteriously attractive than beauty: it is corruption.

—*Octave Mirbeau*

The French port of Dieppe (dee-EPP) lies about 75 miles across the English Channel from Newhaven, England. During peacetime, the ferry was traditionally the most convenient passage between the two places. By the summer of 1942, however, the German army had occupied Dieppe for nearly two years and had deployed a sizable unit of soldiers and ordinance to defend the port against attack. This was no major investment, but merely a garden-variety defensive installation in one of the mid-sized channel ports. At this point Hitler was still winning the war and had not yet fortified the beaches between the towns with obstacles and more complex forces—all that would come later, when they actually prepared for an allied invasion. The British public was getting increasingly impatient with its leadership, clamoring for a "second front" to be launched against the Nazis in addition to the Russian front. However, the British government was divided as to their next move.

Prime Minister Winston Churchill, surrounded by both military and political advisors, wanted to take the offensive and capture territory back from the Germans. One of the ideas kicked around in the war room was a "super raid," an invasion of a port by a massive force. The purpose was to divide the German resources (which would help the Soviets), bring on a massive air battle, and then abandon the port after holding it for no more than one day. One of these super raids, Operation Jubilee, was for raiding Dieppe. Louis Mountbatten, a young cousin of the royal family, had been placed in charge of an allied planning unit called Combined Operations, and he was in charge of Operation Jubilee. This job was quite important, but some of the more experienced commanders considered him a lightweight and believed his appointment more a public relations move by Churchill than a sensible way to tighten the war machine.

Mountbatten never received approval from the chiefs of staff for his raid on Dieppe, although he spent the rest of his life assuring the world he had. The chiefs rejected plans similar to Operation Jubilee, but Mountbatten didn't want to waste an opportunity for personal glory. When Churchill learned of Jubilee's defeat he was in Russia on a diplomatic mission. The news came as a shock, since he didn't know Operation Jubilee was even attempted. However, he did not say that Mountbatten did not have approval for the operation—to say so would expose the incompetence of his personnel. Although the Chiefs of Staff never their gave approval, they didn't seem to mind that an unauthorized Mountbatten led away enough planes, ships and loaded landing craft for a raiding operation.

In the words of historian Brian Villa, the assault party attacked the beach "despite the fact that he did not have either the capital ships or the heavy bombers that alone could have counter-balanced the defenders' firepower and give the attacking force any chance at all." Another question to ask is why the party landed in daylight without any smoke screens to hide from German fire? And why did they advance straight into a fortified harbor rather than land down the undefended beach and come in from the sides or behind? It all seems like a classroom exercise on how to doom a mission, explainable only by Mountbatten's ambition and incompetence, and the blind commitment of Churchill and the royal family to protect Mountbatten from paying the normal price for the reckless abuse of trust and power.

Dieppe was not the only odd moral choice Churchill made. Before the war's end he chose not to relieve the famine-stricken population of Bengal and watched 3-5 million Bengalis die from disease and starvation. More famously, after the allies achieved command over European air space, his bombing crews failed to destroy the railway lines leading to the German death camps. In all, he could have prevented millions of deaths by making a few phone calls, but he just didn't. Mountbatten, having not been stopped or even reprimanded, was eventually promoted to supreme commander of the allied forces in Southeast Asia, gaining the title "Earl of Burma" from the final victory in that region.

At any rate, Operation Jubilee was one of the most costly and embarrassing blunders of the whole war, on either side. No nation understands this better than the Canadians. Out of the 6,000 troops that assaulted the beach that day, most were from the Canadian second division South Saskatchewan regiment, and only a handful made it to the town; 1,700 were killed or wounded and another 1,900 were captured and spent the rest of the war in internment camps. Not one of the Canadians had any previous battle experience. Every tank that landed had to be sacrificed, mainly because their treads were not suited for the Dieppe gravel and simply fell off. Aside from the gravel, there were anti-tank ditches and concrete barriers in plain sight blocking all entrances to the town. We can presume the planners of the attack were familiar with the Normandy coast, yet because of poor planning 33 landing craft never made it past the beach.

Down the beach at a village called Puys (pwee), a flanking Canadian infantry battalion ran into what Allied historians called "bad luck." The German commander had ordered a "practice alert" for his battalion, so the beach defenses were fully manned. The Canadians were met by machinegun fire the moment they stepped from the landing craft. Hand grenades from the cliffs rained down upon those who lived through the first barrage. If Allied intelligence had been involved, they might have created a diversion or at least made sure that this German unit was elsewhere on the day of the raid. As it happened, Mountbatten didn't use intelligence, and his team was completely clueless. To this day Canadians are bitter about the massacre, even though a good share of the blame goes to the Canadian General McNaughton. McNaughton could have refused involvement because there was no evidence of War Cabinet approval, but he simply took Mountbatten's word that everything was a go.

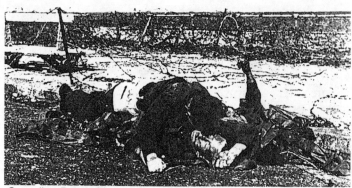

Canadian Dead, Dieppe, August 19. 1942

"There were pieces of human beings littering the beach. There were headless bodies, there were legs, there were arms. And they looked inhuman. ...there were shoes lying around —with feet in them."

—*A Dieppe survivor*

The German casualties were about 600 men and 200 planes. Since the Allies lost only 100 planes, this attrition rate got some favorable mention. For their part the Nazi commanders were somewhat bewildered by the ease by which they had defended the port. But why did the British Government cover up the fact that one of its pet idiots, the picturesque but incompetent Louis Mountbatten, jumped the chain of command and led thousands of soldiers (mostly from another country) into a virtual meat grinder just to put a few laurels on his own head? Their reasons were very clear: If they had admitted that Mountbatten had acted without authority, it would have caused a breach of trust between Britain and Canada, and possibly between Britain and other Commonwealth nations. During the war such a scandal would also badly undermine confidence in Britain's military leadership—a grave concern, to say the least. Furthermore, the scandal could have shaken public confidence in the government itself, particularly because Mountbatten orchestrated this blunder through his royal connections. The method ultimately decided upon to cover up this atrocity was innovative: They called it an experiment.

The disastrous Operation Jubilee was called a "rehearsal for invasion" two years before the invasion of Normandy (Operation Overlord) took place in June 1944. For half a century, command apologists have incessantly aligned the two operations in a direct relationship, as if winning the war was only possible because "valuable lessons" were learned at Dieppe. On the eve of the Normandy invasion, the 3rd Canadian Division was told that "the plan, the preparations, the method and technique" of their new mission was "based on knowledge and experience bought and paid for by the 2nd Canadian division at Dieppe." Mountbatten called Jubilee "one of the great deception operations of the war," suggesting that it misled the Germans into thinking that the invasion was to take place at a major port like Cherbourg or Le Havre—ports capable of handling large-scale troop landings. Of course it would have been foolish to directly attack those ports, but that's a matter of strategic first principles—no one needed a suicide mission at Dieppe to gain such intelligence. Mountbatten swore by the importance of Dieppe for the rest of his life. "I do hope," he wrote in 1973, "the Dieppe boys will have at last understood that without their valiant efforts we could never have had Overlord."

"An outdated or poorly conceived experiment often yields irrelevant data."

—John Campbell

Another alleged lesson of Dieppe was how to jam or

falsely trigger the defensive radar systems the Nazis had placed along the European coastline. Historian John Campbell has carefully examined the developments in radar technology over the course of the war, as well as the strategies and counter-strategies for invasions that followed Jubilee. He discovered that regarding radar, little or no value was placed on Dieppe; no new jamming devices were tried during the mission, no German devices were captured, and the Germans were not tricked into exposing any defense systems that the Allies had not yet encountered.

Historians have also mentioned that Jubilee involved a small force of troops, a tiny clique of generals and a few miles of coastline, while Overlord involved hundreds of thousands of troops, the total involvement of the regional Allied resources, and an unbelievably complex coordination of intelligence, communications and supply transport. One can't plan for surgery on a whale by dissecting a sardine. Another problem is the time lapse: Two years passed between the two operations, and between Dieppe and D-Day the Germans had developed new radar technology and installed massive additional defense systems throughout France. During that two year gap several large-scale amphibious landings occurred all over Europe. Everything worthy of consideration for Normandy was tested after Dieppe. Thick encyclopedias on the Battle of Normandy exist that make no mention of Dieppe. As one historian quipped, if it "was a rehearsal... it certainly wasn't a dress rehearsal."

Mountbatten lived a long and luxurious life, but he never really forgot Dieppe. A year before his death he said to a Canadian TV producer, "[I do not understand] why they wish to go on reveling in the massacres with their martyrism. They [just] want to revel in their misery." Throughout his postwar life he often stated "It is a curious thing, but a fact, that I have been right in everything I have done and said in my life." In 1979, while relaxing on his yacht, a bomb planted by the Irish Republican Army blew Louis Mountbatten to pieces.

The Tragedy of Nicole Wan:
How to Make Malpractice Smell Like a Rose by a Wave of the Experimental Wand

"Iteration and reiteration will be necessary to eradicate the error of the drugging to sleep of the cough reflex, which is the protector of the lungs."
—Chevalier Jackson, MD, in Bronchoesophagology, Philadelphia & London: W.B. Saunders (1950).

Hoi Yan (Nicole) Wan was a 19-year old University of Rochester freshman who died during an air pollution and secondhand smoke study on March 31, 1996. The study began in 1981 and involved the harvesting of lung cells through a procedure called a bronchoscopy. In this procedure, the local anesthetic lidocaine is sprayed down the throat to control gagging while a flexible 7mm-x-40cm bronchoscope is inserted down the subject's windpipe. Ms. Wan was complaining of chest pains, weakness and was coughing blood when she was discharged from the study at Strong Memorial Hospital. Questions remain as to whether the attending physician, Dr. Mark Frampton, was even in attendance; he may have let his intern do the procedures unsupervised. Two hours after her discharge, Wan returned to the hospital's emergency room suffering from a heart attack. She slipped into a coma and died two days later. Her family sued for wrongful death and demanded $100 million while the university floundered for answers. On October 3, 1996, the family and the University jointly announced that an out of court settlement had been reached. The settlement came a few days after the New York State Department of Health found Dr. Mark Frampton guilty of allowing intern Dr. Edgar Geigel to administer four times the maximum dose of lidocaine. Frampton was also found guilty of failing to clearly state the maximum dosages in the study's protocol, violating the stated guidelines, and failing to properly monitor the young woman's condition after the procedure. The finding by the state health department officials did not carry any penalties, but was passed along to the Federal Office for Protection from Research Risks, which can sanction institutions and is conducting its own probe.

The settlement stipulated that the university erect a memorial to Ms. Wan, offer scholarships to Chinese-American students and sponsor an annual lecture on the ethical and safety issues involved in human research. An undisclosed amount of money was agreed upon, described only as "reasonable compensation satisfactory to the Wan family." The Wans did not know their daughter was participating in the study until her hospitalization, and the family is reportedly pushing for a requirement that research volunteers under age 20 have parental consent. In reporting Wan's death, the media referred to the bronchoscopy as an "experiment." Moreover, New York State Health Commissioner Barbara De Buono connected the accident to the research protocol, missing the point that it was not the protocol but the doctors' ineptitude that caused Nicole Wan's death. Both of these misinterpretations blur the seriousness of Dr. Frampton's and Dr. Geigel's error and serve to whitewash the social implications of the tragedy. Like the Dieppe calamity, this tragedy has remained an experiment gone wrong in the public consciousness.

Lidocaine has been used since 1946 and is hardly an experimental drug. According to Dorland's Medical

Dictionary, bronchoscopies have been practiced since 1898. The tissue sampling Nicole Wan died from was part of a long-term study of the effects of air pollution on the U.S. population. The tissue biopsy is itself virtually an ancient procedure, dating back to the invention of the microscope in the 1850's. This means that Nicole Wan's fatal experience at Strong Memorial Hospital had no experimental features—she underwent an entirely routine procedure. The recording of data was to begin when the lung cells reached the laboratory, and even at that point the word "experiment" would be a bit of a stretch. Frampton and company know all about lidocaine, bronchoscopies and biopsies because they're physicians and lung specialists, and not because they read a particular protocol that described the harvesting of lung tissues from study volunteers.

In April '96 a spokesperson for the University of Rochester said that Dr. Geigel had performed "more than 100 bronchoscopies without incident" before the case of Nicole Wan. So why did he forget such basics as the maximum safe dosage of lidocaine and the need for careful observation after administering the drug to a patient? Why did he disregard Nicole's complaints of chest pain and weakness? Why didn't her coughing up blood mean anything to him? Let's consider some possibilities:

"The safety and effectiveness of lidocaine depends on proper dosage, adequate precautions and readiness for emergencies."
—Physicians' Desk Reference,
49th edition (1995), page 580.

Since Ms. Wan's death the author has interviewed one man and one young woman who volunteered for the same study in Philadelphia and Boston. Both said that the procedure went smoothly and that it seemed like easy cash. I myself have been intubated for a stomach research study that used lidocaine. The anesthetic was no big deal. The doctor doing the procedure would stop whenever I gagged on the tube and ask if I was OK.

Doctors in the U.S. are usually not the elite, wealthy, professionally independent operators they are commonly believed to be. Today most are simply the employees of hospitals. Large chains of hospitals in the U.S. are now owned by investment groups, and are managed not by physicians, but by people holding business degrees. Foreigners who seek treatment here often express disgust with the rushed, impersonal demeanor of American doctors. The medical profession has been bastardized by big business: The typical physician is badly overworked, and the salesmanship of pharmaceutical firms and the constraints of "managed care" heavily influence his decisions. But a few doctors are still the wise, well-rested and deeply caring super-people who we all want at our bedside in times of crisis; these are also the ones the average person cannot afford.

Suppose that a young woman in that same study had returned to that same hospital with a foreign object lodged in her esophagus; say she has a few wealthy relatives at her side, summoning their professional friends on cell phones and bearing the full compliment of insurance ID cards; she may well be seen by the same doctor, and she may need a bronchoscopy. However, in such a case, the doc would know in his bones that if he made the smallest mistake or if his conduct was less than perfect, the payback would be swift and sure. He would devote extra time to her and would be more demanding of his support staff.

A Mountbatten could expect such treatment, but Nicole was not in his social class. She was just a guinea pig, someone strapped for cash who was essentially renting her own body in an honorable but, to some, an undesirable manner. This was not someone with a lawyer at her beck and call. Harvesting her lung cells was a monotonous schlep-job for the doctor. In Wan's case they understood their conduct would not be carefully monitored. The effects of their carelessness were bound to emerge in the case of a weaker patient, but Dr. Frampton and Dr. Geigel, not unlike Mountbatten, suffered no serious consequences. One might argue that the doctors should have been prosecuted as criminals (and a few doctors have said so off the record), but the worst they could ever expect are long, easy practices in prison infirmaries, or some other duty out of the fast lane. As it happens, Frampton is still practicing and experimenting at Rochester, and Geigel was last spotted practicing in the Miami area.

The Wan out-of-court settlement not only sidesteps the doctors' carelessness, but also smacks of false sympathy and concern. This is what galls me the most: The University of Rochester took advantage of Nicole Wan's vulnerable position as a cash-strapped student, then easily got itself off the hook because of her family's very understandable wish to put the whole tragedy behind them. Any doctors who perform bronchoscopies without knowing everything about lidocaine and its dangers are butchers and slobs who should be run out of the profession on a rail. Yet these two, Frampton and Geigel, have been publicly excused.

We have seen one real battle experiment, Guernica, and looked at how its true motives were later denied. The pure military blunder of Dieppe was excused on the shabby argument that it had provided valuable lessons, as if it were an experiment. Finally, the accidental death of a healthy young woman by blundering doctors was played in the media as the unforeseen result of an experiment, a line that clouded the truth of malpractice, not unlike the

Dieppe apologists. In wartime and in peacetime, in battle and in medicine, amoral actions and mistakes of incompetence are sometimes sugarcoated with the spin that the failed action actually served the best interests of humanity, but these ends never justify the means.

For Further Reading:

Brian L. Villa, *Unauthorized Action: Mountbatten and the Dieppe Raid.* Toronto: Oxford University Press, 1989.

John P. Campbell, *Dieppe Revisited: A Documentary Investigation.* Toronto and London: Frank Cass Publishers, 1993.

Personal Library Publishers, *Echoes of Disaster: Dieppe 1942.* Toronto: Personal Library, 1979

Dorothy Legarreta, *The Guernica Generation: Basque Refugee Children of the Spanish Civil War.* Reno: University of Nevada Press, 1984.

Anthony Beevor, *The Spanish Civil War.* London: Orbis, 1982.

Gordon Thomas and Max Morgan Witts, *Guernica: the Crucible of WW2.* New York: Stein & Day, 1975.

Herbert R. Southworth, "Guernica." In James W. Cortada, ed., *Historical Dictionary of the Spanish Civil War 1936-1939.* Westport and London: Greenwood, 1982.

The Guinea Pig Strike at PENN, June 1935
BY ROBERT HELMS

*"It is to the problem of the capture, selection, care, and train-
ing of good healthy human guinea pigs, if I may use a trite
phrase, that I would invite your attention."*
—*Dr. William Osler Abbott, 1939*

In 1931, gastroenterologist William Osler Abbott
(1902-1943) was developing faster techniques for "intubating the human intestine from mouth to rectum" while
he was an instructor at the Hospital of the University of
Pennsylvania. This research perfected the use of the
"Miller-Abbot tube" which, in its day, was an important
aid in the treatment of stomach and intestinal disorders.

Having dismissed the idea of intubating laboratory
dogs as "a waste of time," he sought two-legged volunteers
to swallow a flexible 12-foot double-lumen tube with a
rubber balloon attached to it. The balloon was inflated
inside the intestine, and then the subject was X-rayed with
a device called a fluoroscope. Abbott swallowed the tubes
himself till he was "sick at the sight of them," he said in a
speech before the Charaka Club of New York in February,
1939. The tube, by the way, was removed back through
the mouth, while earlier tubes traveled on a one-way street
out the back door. As he continued the research, he failed
to find willing patients in the hospital wards, so he went
to an employment bureau in the city. The agent there
refused to send men to him after learning exactly what the
job involved. Abbott then got the wives of some of his
friends to stand on the South Street Bridge (which crosses
the Schuylkill River adjacent to the PENN campus) and
hand out leaflets to poor people offering $2 per day for a
job at the hospital. This method was also fruitless. At his

secretary's suggestion, he decided to use a black janitor from the hospital floor named Harry to recruit healthy subjects. They were to appear at the door of the lab at 8:30 in the morning, and Harry got fifty cents for each one that came "sober and in a fasting state."

At this point in Abbott's fascinating narrative, he actually gives the name of the first person to respond to Harry's call. It was Flip Lawall, "tall, broad-shouldered, black as the ace of spades, and by profession a lightweight prize fighter," who fought at the Arena at 46th & Market Streets (now long gone), about a mile from the university. Many other black men followed, and soon Abbott had them paired and scheduled weeks in advance, "giving a spacing that allowed of fluoroscopy without too frequent exposures." Here the good doc demonstrates that he understood the risks involved in the radiation, but nowhere does he say that he conveyed this knowledge to Flip and the other recruits, who would sometimes stretch out under the trees in the medical school's botanical gardens, swallowing long coils of tubing "to the scandal of the neighborhood." What seems to have been most important was that the guinea pigs were in good supply for a while.

As every recruiter of human subjects discovers, they're not all perfect. Dr. Abbott complains that "Harry slipped in an epileptic who flew into a convulsion and bit off a wonderfully complicated tube I had spent hours devising." Luckily the lower end was not far from his rectum, so that the lost three yards were soon recovered. Another, more remarkable episode was when he was intubating the duodenum of a guy named "Jim" with the guidance of his fluoroscope when he recognized a .38 caliber revolver bullet in the muscle surrounding the man's spinal column. Jim "grinned sheepishly" and explained that his sweetheart had shot him the night before when he dropped in to see her, unaware that she'd spotted him with another woman that same evening. "Such events led me to wish at times that I could keep my animals in metabolism cages," the gut doctor reflected. He also commented that "they stole all the inkwells and pens from the dispensary."

"I'm sure my animals had a larger intake of corn liquor, pork chops, and chewing tobacco than the white rats in the medical school, but at least they were humans ...."
—Dr. W. Osler Abbott, 1939

Harry was getting the men into the gastroenterology ward regularly and on time, and all was well when Abbott was scheduled to exhibit his state-of-the-art intubations before the 86th Annual Convention of the American Medical Association (AMA), held June 10-14, 1935 at the Ambassador Hotel in Atlantic City, New Jersey. Abbott describes an emerging pattern of men who "sheepishly refused" their payment, asking to be paid a day or two later instead. This did not interfere with the plans for the big presentation. "It was arranged that two subjects a day would appear at the Atlantic City Hospital in time to be intubated under the fluoroscope and brought to the convention hall booth by 9:00 AM. A special expense account and a liberal bonus was arranged."

At 1:30 PM, on a certain day less than a week before the convention, Dr. Abbott was taken by surprise:

> ...the whole crowd went on strike together. Double the pay or no demonstration was the demand. That was a bad few minutes for me. No dogs, cats, rats, or rabbits that I had ever handled had done this, but there was one opening left. At 2 o'clock the last examination of the Spring term, third year obstetrics, was due to begin. I left the Black delegation sitting and sprinted for the Medical School. As the stu-

dents gathered, I gave them an impassioned appeal for volunteers, offered the pay of my striking black-amoors, and in five minutes a shipment of scab labor had signed up. That would have made any factory foreman green with envy. Thereupon I returned to the committee, and, the National Labor Relations Board being as yet unborn, I had the pleasure of indulging in a little old-fashioned capitalism. I fired the whole lot of them, lock, stock, and barrel. The exhibit went off like clockwork. The volunteers from the third year class stood up to those tubes like veterans of the line.

The presentation at Atlantic City was called "Exhibit on the Small Intestine," and it won a "Special Certificate of Honor" from the AMA as well as other prizes, a major career achievment for Abbott.

Let us observe that Dr. Abbott did not regard his human subjects as equal partners in the research process. Indeed, he likened them to animals, and he viewed them as inferiors both as men of color and as members of the working class. Later that year, he stated that Harry the janitor confided in him about Flip Lawall and his "pure racket." Lawall would supposedly beat up any guinea pig who arrived late and took a cut of each man's pay. This was stated as the reason why some of the men asked to be paid at odd hours.

As is so often the case when an employer replaces reliable workers with scab labor, the eloquent doctor felt the loss of their assistance and tried to find them again in October of the same year. "Those boys may have been short on morals but they were long in gut," he quipped. But Flip was by then no longer available. He had been convicted of a rape and was starting a 10-year stretch in the penetentiary. Abbott lamented the idleness of his star guinea pig:

> I often passed those grim walls and thought of the many feet of well-trained intestine lying fallow, inexorably removed from the service of humanity. In the millenium perhaps the whole will no longer have to suffer for the part, and the bar association may devise a means of incarcerating only the offending organ thereby leaving the entrails at large, so to speak.

The narrative continues with the shrewd tube-twister switching to the practice of advertising in the two major city newspapers as follows: "Wanted: healthy adult men (or women) to act as subjects in medical experiments. Fifty cents per hour, one day in two weeks. Apply 1:30 PM, tomorrow, room 323, Hospital of the University of Pennsylvania." It's my impression that Abbott supplies us with the times of day here and earlier when the strike occured (both 1:30 PM) so as to illustrate himself as a strategist returning with an effective counter-movement. He was inundated with applicants, and after scaring away a large portion of them with thickly-laid descriptions of the job, and how one could earn as much as $1.50 per hour by swallowing three tubes at once, he finished with a list of 78 die-hards who still wanted in. From these, he was to pick twelve. Payment was to be made when the guinea pig signed a document accepting all risks involved and acknowledged that the process was an experiment.

For all of his character defects, Dr. Abbott certainly was fascinated with his experimental subjects, and he asked the new recruits a long list of questions so that he could get a good, even sample of the population—of the white population, that is. His very thorough description mentions no blacks, and turns strikingly sympathetic as he asks each applicant why they had come:

> ...in that afternoon I learned a great truth about humanity and Economic reverses. There were only five in that whole assembly who were destitute or on relief. Every other one was feeling the pinch of depression and fighting to keep off relief at any cost. It was a heroic little army fighting for self respect in an age of itching palms. Almost all were fathers or mothers of families that could just barely get along. Almost all had some sort of part-time job with which they could eke out a living by extra work. There was a high proportion of elderly who could not get jobs because the workmen's compensation laws hung over the heads of possible employers... In the end I had a list of many more than I could use, mainly married men and women whose children needed that pair of shoes that a meager wage would not buy... That was a revolution. The whole aspect of things had changed. There was no more paying one man to get another in at the appointed time. They were always on hand. There was no more debating with myself whether the smell of stale liquor on the breath was strong enough to warrant abandoning the experiment. There was in fact a growing spirit of pride in the game and loyalty to the department that was fascinating to watch.

These last remarks are evidence of the triumphant and vindictive pleasure the researcher took in foiling the organizing efforts of his former subjects, and also of his joy in replacing his black workers with whites.

When we examine the doctor's narrative of the strike led by the prizefighter Flip Lawall, we find a transparent historical distortion from his own self-interested viewpoint, aside from the more obvious racism that skews his speech. Lawall apparently made the sensible calculation that the eve of the presentation at Atlantic City was a good time to present the demands of his tiny union. One would also assume that the guinea pigs were not eager to be placed on display like circus animals in some demonstration booth at a medical convention, especially given the racial aspect of the scene.

Another noticeable omission occurs when Dr. Abbott fails to state the rate of his "special expense account" and the amount of the "liberal bonus" that he says he offered to the subjects. He gives exact sums at every other point where he discussed payments to subjects. Also suspicious is the assertion that Lawall was racketeering when he collected funds from the men at pay time, if indeed he collected any. Considering he demanded higher pay on the other subjects' behalf, it could be he was collecting union membership dues and that some of the men were trying to avoid making the payments, as is sometimes the case in an organizing drive. Here again the doctor-employer fails to state the amount of the "cut of each man's profits" that Flip Lawall allegedly extorted prior to the strike in 1935.

The available information indicates that the strike involved not less than eight guinea pigs, but it may have been many more than that. Abbott states that "the whole crew" walked together, and he makes it perfectly clear that all of them were black. We have no biographical information on Lawall beyond Abbott's testimony, but what we do have makes us wonder: Was his rape conviction entirely legitimate, or was it helped along by the fighter's labor activism?

For all his shortcomings, when viewed some sixty years in hindsight, Abbott is remembered fondly by his peers in medicine. He died of myelogenous leukemia at age forty-one, only eight years after the guinea pig strike.

I find his writing so eminently quotable that it's not easy for me to hate him, either. Abbott's purpose in writing his anecdotal speech to the Charaka Club (aside from presenting a stand-up racist comedy act) was to argue that it made more sense for researchers and medical school faculty to employ reliable human subjects than to piece their trials and demonstrations together with animals and with hospital patients without their consent.

> There are those willing subjects who are glad to help by being shown off, and there are the stupid ones who think a demonstration is a treatment, but with voluntary professional subjects knowing what it is all about, from whom nothing need be hidden (save perhaps in the field of habit-forming drugs), before whom one can talk freely to the students, everything is easier. This is an answer to the comment made by many, first, that one cannot hire voluntary subjects, next that they cannot be controlled, and finally that the whole thing is impractical.

The overall meaning that this researcher conveys is that he loves us and needs us, so long as we know our place. Let all guinea pigs ponder this and disobey—if they dare, and only if they stick together.

Sources:
Susan E. Lederer, *Subjected to Science: Human Experimentation in America before the Second World War.* Baltimore: Johns Hopkins University Press, 1995. Pp. 121-123

W. Osler Abbott, "The Problem of the Professional Guinea Pig," *Proceedings of the Charaka Club*, 1941, 10, 249-60.

T. Grier Miller and W. Osler Abbott, "Intestinal Intubation: A Practical Technique," *American Journal of Medical Science*, 1934, 187, 595-99.

William C. Stadie, "William Osler Abbott," *Transactions of the Association of American Physicians*, 1944, 58, 7-9.
AMA, "Report of the A[tlantic] C[ity] Conference," *Journal of the American Medical Association*, 1935, July issues.

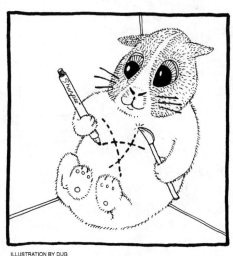

ILLUSTRATION BY DUG

Jaundice, Art, and Death in New Haven, 1944-45

BY ROBERT HELMS

In 1940 President Franklin Roosevelt signed a new law that legally defined noncombatant service and conscientious objectors (CO's). The law helped pacifists avoid a repetition of the brutality they experienced during WWI, and also helped the government gain a healthy crop of volunteer human guinea pigs. In a rare departure from the widespread pattern of underground recruitment and casual (if not brutal) mistreatment, the pacifist research subjects of WWII were well-organized and self-respecting U.S. citizens. The general public also regarded these subjects with a measure of respect.

The task of running the new programs of the Civilian Public Service (CPS) was given to administrative bodies from the three "peace churches": the American Friends Service Committee (AFSC), the Brethren Service Committee, and the Mennonite Central Committee. They also received help from the Unitarian Service Committee, and an advisory organization called the National Service Board for Religious Objectors. The AFSC, organized by Quakers, was in charge of the largest portion of the CPS structure.

The way it worked was any draft-age man who could successfully prove he held a bona fide religious principle for not fighting could register as a CO and be classified as "4-E." An authorized CO would then receive a form letter from the President entitled *Order to Report for Work of National Importance*. The letter gave a time and date for the CO to report to one of the various CPS camps established around the country. Eventually 151 of these camps were established, housing almost 12,000 men. Some camps served as administrative offices for smaller sites that were scattered around a given region.

Labor at most CPS camps included tasks like taking care of the elderly and disabled, maintaining roads and irrigation systems, and working for the forest service. Life was dull and the work was very hard, so it's no small wonder there were so many takers when literature was circulated to recruit volunteer guinea pigs. Over the course of the war, about 1,000 of the CPS men volunteered to serve as subjects in over 50 medical experiments, while others were assigned to the guinea pig units as technicians and nursing staff.

The CPS guinea pigs gained substantial credibility and respect in the mainstream media. As one promotional pamphlet quotes from the *Sioux City Tribune-Journal*:

> In any nation at war, it is so customary to glorify deeds of fighting men that it is generally assumed there is no other form of heroism than facing danger and death on the fighting front... Considering this situation, there seems reason to say a word of commendation for the CO's who are serving as voluntary guinea pigs... They should certainly get credit in the public thinking for what they are doing for the country and its citizens.

Even Major General Lewis Hershey, the selective service director whose job it was to punish those who refused to fight, singled out the lab rats for special praise:

> The new type of [CPS] projects, particularly the so-called 'guinea pig' experiments, are not only of national importance but of the widest humanitarian service. They will help to build up increasing respect for the courage and the seriousness of the

conscientious objectors' convictions.

The general was right. But while nothing like the mass-murders in the guise of research occurring on the Axis side, the CPS research still put the healthy volunteer at more risk than would be acceptable by today's research standards. The acceptable risk level in CPS research could be roughly compared to the demands that would later be exacted from prison inmate volunteers in postwar America.

Unlike civilian prison experiments and military medical atrocities, the CPS volunteer guinea pigs were free to develop their own culture and comradeship through publishing their own newsletters and giving outside press interviews. These sources also provide historians with an enormous amount of contemporary information on top of the voluminous records preserved by the AFSC. For instance, there are unmistakable patterns in the demographics of the CPS volunteers, unless my research accidentally hit upon only well-educated white men with connections to liberal religious denominations and historic "peace churches." However, they served without pay or provisions for their dependants and received no workmen's compensation or insurance; it must be emphasized that by no stretch of the imagination were the conscientious objectors afforded any of the benefits received by regular GI's.

The research with CPS volunteers involved three major areas: disease, nutrition, and exposure to abnormal environments. The research attempted to investigate wartime problems with both military and civilian populations. The problems included typhus, famine, prolonged malnutrition, and risks encountered by heavy troop concentrations in malaria-infested areas. World War II also presented special problems, like jeopardy to body and mind resulting from high-altitude flying and shipwrecks at sea.

Infectious hepatitis is caused by a virus that inflames the liver. Its older name is jaundice, and it often causes the skin of its sufferers to turn yellow. The disease is seldom fatal but always extremely debilitating, and takes at least two months under medical care for it to fully run its course. An epidemic may occur whenever large numbers of people are brought together for an extended period without sufficient sanitation, such as in army, refugee or concentration camps. Children and young adults are the most vulnerable. Beyond its normal existence, the disease was a particular problem for the U.S. military in WWII because it infected the blood supply; thousands of cases are believed to have resulted from jaundice-contaminated Yellow Fever vaccines that were given to great numbers of civilians and military personnel.

In 1943 the CPS program began recruiting volunteers for experiments aimed at learning more about how the virus spreads. These experiments were conducted at two hospitals in Philadelphia and two in New Haven, Connecticut, and used at least 154 CPS men as subjects. The CPS guinea pigs on duty were given "waste matter from persons with Jaundice" (presumably feces mixed into the volunteers' food or water), and 3 of every 5 men contracted the disease. This means that over 90 of them were flat on their backs with hepatitis for 7 to 9 weeks, and different groups of these volunteers were given different medication diets to see what worked better against the disease. Needless to say, this study was very hazardous and demanding, and there probably were some great jokes about the food.

According to contemporary reports the experiment itself was a success. It was determined that the pathogen was indeed a virus, that jaundice was a "filth disease," and that there were a few different varieties. Preventive measures and new treatments were developed, and the Pentagon would now be able to heal more afflicted troops in less time and get them back on the battlefield.

One source of information for the experiences of the CPS guinea pigs is the newsletter they created through the Yale University Medical School in New Haven called *The Guinea Gazette.** Produced around the end of 1944 with amusing illustrations by David H. Miller and Tom Steger, the 11-page publication began during the incubation period of the disease, about a month after the 27-man subject group was formed. While waiting for the disease to incubate, the jaundice men worked at hospital jobs and with the Connecticut Forest Service. During the incubation, they were set up in a dormitory on the Yale campus, and as symptoms appeared they were placed in the isolation unit at the Yale hospital.

Artist Thomas Steger's career went far beyond the few small cartoons he doodled in *The Guinea Gazette.* He was recruited from the CPS camp at Coshocton, Indiana, where he had already done a mural at the Merom Institute. *The Guinea Gazette* states that during the incubation, Steger was asked to do a series of paintings called *The History of Epidemiology in New Haven*, which were to hang in a conference room at Yale's Sterling Hall of Medicine.

One of the other men was assigned to the medical school's animal quarters, which housed about 1,500 mice and 50 monkeys with poliomyelitis. He had to clean the cages and was told ahead of time that he'd need special work clothes because "the smell stays in your clothes and makes you offensive to society." Without identifying him, his fellow subjects tease him in the newsletter about how

---

* Its title seems to have been intended to distinguish it from another CPS newsletter, *The Guinea Pig Gazette*, started by lab rats doing nutrition experiments at the University of Minnesota in May, 1943.

he enjoys the company of the two chimpanzees:

> He waxes quite eloquent about them. Walking hand-in-hand to find a banana; cuddling close and whispering sweet nothings in an ear... we never get quite straight who whispered what to whom... and I've been under the impression that hepatitis was a disease of the liver!

The human guinea pig in question really did enjoy tending to the needs of his non-human colleagues. He describes his job on the "Mouspital" in the Gazette as follows:

> "My duties consist of keeping the mice in feed and water, and doing their general housekeeping, inspecting the pens daily for untimely sick or dead mice, and recording the pregnancies and litters...
>
> "The mice are well-behaved, in a mousy sort of way. The senile and breeders are in separate wards, while in the experimental section are those being used in current experiments. Two of the experiments at present are in sex hormones and tumor research.
>
> "Although my nose has learned to ignore the powerful odor, I am most unpopular in the dining hall. Such is the price of being a successful mouspitalitarian."

The Death of Warren Dugan (1918-1945)

"There have been 9 or 10 deaths of CPS assignees which have been attributed in some manner or other to their assigned work."

-Dr. John R. Paul, Yale Medical School,
November 7, 1945

A few of the CO's involved with the medical research were employed as medical technicians. An unusual accident took the life of Warren Gilbert Dugan, a 27 year-old mechanical engineer who had non-medical laboratory experience prior to his assignment at CPS Camp #140, the Connecticut Jaundice Unit at Yale. One of his jobs at Yale was to use a centrifuge to prepare doses of poliomyelitis for polio-infected monkeys. He seems to have been well trained and supervised, but something still went wrong. On August 17, 1945, he began showing symptoms of polio, but did not seek medical attention until the 24th. He was then diagnosed and treated for the disease, but his infection was so strong that he died two days later.

Warren was the bright, rebellious son of a Unitarian family in Illinois. His stepfather was a state senator from Massachusetts, his mom an artist, his dad a newspaper editor. He was educated at Antioch and Harvard. He was drafted in March 1943, became a CO and was first given work in psychiatric hospitals. He applied at Yale, was taken on staff in October 1944, and was seen to be "a careful and conscientious worker." The lab worker's death was immediately publicized as "probably" the result of a laboratory infection. The physician in charge of the polio experiments and who also treated Dugan came across only one other such accident four years prior to this incident.

Dugan was not a guinea pig, and had signed no waiver against possible injury or death, so he qualified for workman's compensation. The AFSC paid for his funeral, and there was some discussion of a Carnegie Medal in acknowledgment of his pacifist work. There was even a bill introduced to Congress asking for death benefits to follow from his sacrifice. A plaque was placed in Yale's medical library, where it probably remains today.

Warren was married just 13 months before he died.

His widow, Doris, studied Music Education and lived in New Haven with her husband. The death was widely reported in the press. Fellow CPS volunteer Norman Whitney said that Warren had given his life "as heroically and sacrificially as any other." Another fellow worker stated, "he did, in reality, lay down his life that others might live. There is no better example of the pacifist answer to the militarist."

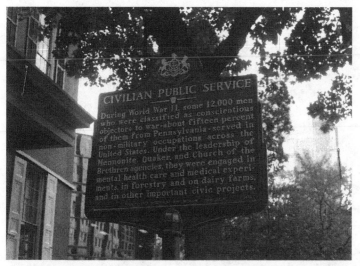

Plaque outside the Philadelphia Friends Center Photo by Robert Helms

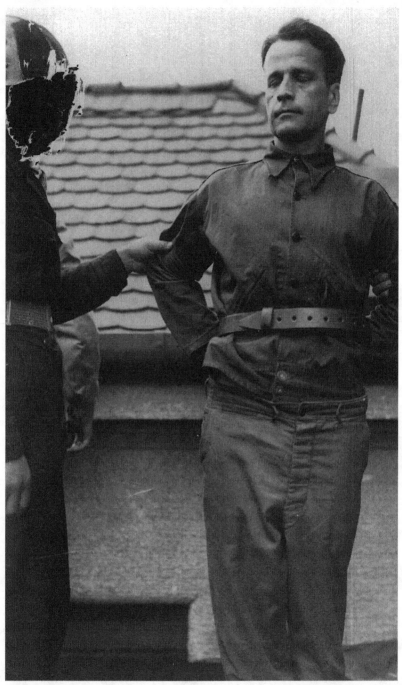

Waldemar Hoven, Captain, Waffen SS. Chief Doctor of Buchenwald Concentration Camp about to be hanged at Landsberg Prison on June 2, 1948. (National Archives Photo)

The Concentration Camp at Natzweiler-Le Struthof, Past and Present

BY ROBERT HELMS

Christmas Eve, 1996 was not the right weekend to be driving around in the French Alps, but one doesn't get to see Alsace every day. As we drove halfway across the country the sky couldn't make up its freezing mind whether we deserved snow or sleet. As night fell it settled on an icy rain and we settled in at a hotel in Strasbourg. When I asked about the old concentration camp, the clerk said that the roads would be too dangerous. She had been there and assured us that any precipitation we saw in the city would be worse at Le Struthof. We talked about it and narrowly agreed among ourselves that it was worth the risk.

The next morning my bones were cold as we approached the camp because of a problem with the car's heating system. I hadn't really dressed for the weather, which just made things worse. The narrow road snaked upward through a heavy fog. Ice had formed on the branches of the high pines alongside the road, making them droop down and appear rounded and surreal. It was a holiday, so my three friends and I were the only people to visit the camp in this horrible weather. The two staffers seemed surprised to see us as we paid and walked through a gate made of heavy wooden poles. As a human guinea pig, I was interested in the camp as the site of deadly experiments conducted by Nazi doctors during WWII.

Natzweiler and Le Struthof are the two nearby villages that give the concentration camp its name. Although small in comparison with other camps, it held 7,000-8,000 deportees and had eighteen satellite work camps called *kommandos* that contained an additional 14,000 prisoners. The weather on the day of our visit was perfect for reminding us of the freezing alpine winters endured by the prisoners doing hard labor in inadequate clothing; countless prisoners died from this alone. It was also one of the few camps that received captured politicals, who had their backs marked with an "NN," the German abbreviation for "Night & Fog." These special prisoners were *maquisards*—guerilla fighters and other resistance members from France, Belgium and Holland. They were completely isolated, even within the camp, and quickly and secretly exterminated. Inmates met their ends by hanging, gassing, working to death in an SS granite quarry, or through fatal experiments.

The medical college at Strasbourg University was about 40 minutes away. This college was one of the centers of the Ancestral Hereditary Society, or *Das Ahnenerbe*, a research institute that produced much of the pseudo-scientific justifications for Nazi ethnocentrism. Dr. August Hirt, an anatomist and an SS captain, was a high-ranking official in Das Ahnenerbe. He controlled about a dozen Natzweiler buildings that housed an infirmary, experimental research labs, holding rooms for human guinea pigs after they'd been used, an autopsy room, a gas chamber, and four crematory ovens. There was, and still is, an outdoor gallows where they would hang troublemakers in front other inmates. The SS medical scene was full of mediocre and downright terrible scientists, which is not surprising when one considers how many Jewish, leftist, or otherwise unacceptable persons the Nazi plan had driven out of the field. Dr. Hirt, however, was one of the very few SS medical murderers who had very distinguished professional credentials. Hirt had been a leading professor of anatomy for many years and authored a textbook on anatomy that is still used by some medical colleges—a fact rather disturbing to some of those in the know. It should be said, however, that a great deal of the research leading to his distinction was done in collaboration with a Jewish scientist who later disappeared from Hirt's curriculum vitae.

August Hirt is notorious for murdering some 115 persons to supply material for a "skull collection" housed at Strasbourg University. The idea was to have the skull features from the various ethnicities of the world on record and displayed before the SS exterminated the populations. Most of the people selected for collection material were Jews (79 men, 30 women), as well as two Poles and four Asians. The end of the war neared before this work was completed, and with the camp in danger of capture Hirt executed all of the subjects and ordered their bodies destroyed. The cadavers were not entirely destroyed, however, and after the war 16 entire bodies and the anatomical parts from 70 other Natzweiler inmate cadavers were found preserved in formaldehyde. Photographs of these heavily dissected remains were presented as evidence in the Nuremberg trials of the Nazi doctors.

Another experiment-atrocity that took place under Hirt's supervision was supposedly intended to find better ways to treat burns caused by mustard gas. The experiments he sold to the army had virtually no scientific merit, but it kept the doctor funded and busy until the end of the war. Jews, Russians, Gypsies and Poles were asked to volunteer for the experiments and were even offered money and freedom, but none stepped forward. Around 150 of them were used anyway. After the war, a captured orderly named Ferdinand Holl described the procedures:

> A drop of the liquid was made to fall upon the forearms of the experimental subjects. Then the people had to stand there for some time until the liquid evaporated. 24 to 36 hours later, severe burns

appeared on the entire body. I myself recorded 30 persons being treated this way, with seven cases of death following.

At least 50 of the subjects died in horrible pain from internal burns to vital organs. The others became ill and went blind, so they were sent out for extermination. The reader may be pleased to learn that by accident the doctor caught a whiff of the stuff himself and had to spend time recovering in a hospital. The salves that were concocted by Hirt's team failed in all tests, and no beneficial treatment was ever devised for use by the Nazi military. The anatomist committed suicide in May 1945.

The small museum in one of the former barracks had models of the original layout, maps showing the locations of the satellite camps, and even the old wooden racks where the inmates slept on filthy straw. It also holds numerous photographs of the remains of the human guinea pigs found at Natzweiler after the deserted camp was liberated. It was extremely cold, and since I wasn't really dressed for it, the ice, rain and fog added all I needed to get the feeling of the place. The museum's literature in English is badly translated, and all of it is brief and lacking in photos.

Our friend Michel did the driving that morning. He spent two years in the French army rebuilding the German infrastructure, and had been to Natzweiler in 1960 as a driver for VIP's visiting the site. Along with a few war-related stories, he pointed out some major changes in the camp since his last visit in 1960.

Twice his crew uncovered subterranean passageways with their bulldozers while rebuilding roads near Baden-Baden. Inside each passageway they found about twenty shriveled corpses, just skin and bones, sort of like mummies hung from the napes of their necks on meat hooks.

The ends of the passageways had been walled up. In each case Michel went down to get a look at the bodies and then notified his superiors. They in turn called the German police, who were at the time under French supervision. Michel didn't investigate the matter, but he later heard that the forty-odd cadavers were thought to be German dissidents, murdered by the Third Reich before the war.

Another time, Michel had to drive some high-ranking officials around the Dachau concentration camp, which lies adjacent to a small town bearing the same name. In spite of his being very tired, he found himself unable to remain overnight in the town or even to stop for a drink. He was well aware that this was the earliest of the camps, and that before and throughout the war, despite feeble denials, every person in that town knew exactly what was happening.

The end of the war did not see the end of fascism at Natzweiler. On the night of May 12, 1976, neo-Nazis torched several buildings, including all of the labs and holding rooms. Stones with the names of other death camps now mark the empty plots; Natzweiler inmates were transferred to these camps in 1944 as the allies approached. All of the towers and barbed wire fences still stand, as well as a monument and a cemetery of several thousand graves.

Strasbourg has the second largest Jewish community in France, second only to Paris, and like everywhere else people in Strasbourg are remembering the 50th anniversary of the 1947 "Doctor Trial" at Nuremberg. German Jewish doctors associated with major chemical firms have recently made ovations with French Holocaust remembrance organizations. On their own initiative they orchestrated an event at the Strasbourg Jewish cemetery, and invited survivors, relatives of the dead, and prominent rabbis.

Then in early December, 1997, the physicians installed a plaque on the German side of a bridge crossing the Rhine. The plaque commemorates the dead guinea pigs of the Third Reich. It would have made more sense to install the plaque on the French side, but the doctors seemed to be in a rush to get the thing up, and the decentralized German system handles such matters locally and thus more quickly than the French bureaucracy. I would have provided my readers with a photograph of the plaque, but along with everything else in Alsace that day, it was covered with snow.

For Further Reading:

Frederick H. Kasten, "Unethical Nazi Medicine in Annexed Alsace-Lorriane: The Strange Case of Nazi Anatomist Dr. August Hirt" (in *Historians & Archivists: Essays in Modern German History & Archival Policy*. G. O. Kent, editor, Fairfax, Virginia: University Press, 1991).

The Unspeakable Crimes Of Unit 731

BY PHILLIPE PONS

(Reprinted with permission from *Le Monde*, February 3, 1997. Translated by Robert Helms.)

From 1938 to 1945, the Japanese engaged in bacteriological experiments on human guinea pigs in occupied China. The *Le Monde* correspondent in Manchuria has investigated these yet unpunished atrocities. Covered up by Washington, Tokyo still refuses to acknowledge the facts.

Like resurgent grass on ravaged earth, the town has engulfed the ruins among its buildings. Some sections of wall, a few gutted buildings, the chimneys of incinerators stand here and there on the six square kilometers which could have been some sort of military base. On the railroad track today, merchandise rolls past. Fang Zhen Yu remembers: It was in 1941. He was nineteen years old and he was detained in the camp. Punished, he was sick in a cell, where he looked out on the trains:

> A full load of 'merchandise' arrived. Some men came out of it with their hands tied together. There were more than a hundred of them. Some of them had blond hair. We were a crew of a thousand Chinese employed in what we thought to be a 'water purification center.' We had to transport a lot of food to the 'laboratory.' Sometimes, we would hear harrowing shrieks coming from it. One day, in the dead of winter, I saw a man, completely nude, tied to a post. He was hosed down with water. The water instantly froze on his body, which seemed glazed...

107

It was not so much on the battlefields as here, 20 kilometers south of Harbin in the heart of Manchuria, that the most heinous crimes of World War II's "Asian Theater" took place: Unit 731 proceeded, on a grand scale, with biological experiments and vivisection on human guinea pigs (prisoners from China, Korea, Russia, and perhaps Britain and Holland) in order to equip the Japanese with bacteriological weapons. At the lowest estimate, 3,000 victims (men, women and children) disappeared in the incinerators of the Japanese "death camp."

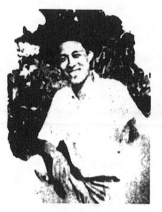 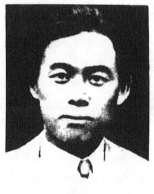

Two Chinese victims of Unit 731 BW experiments

In the little museum of Pingfang, opened in 1982, stands a model of what was once the immense complex (70 buildings) of Unit 731. Behind the long 2-story edifice of the administration building, there was a square structure made up of the prison and the "laboratories." The doors of the cells were fitted with a window through which the prisoners would put their arms to receive injections. The cells were clean and the guinea pigs, who could be as many as one thousand at a time, were treated well, until they became the subjects of experiments. The lodging for 3,000 Japanese (doctors, lab assistants, nurses, and soldiers) was flanked by a Shinto temple. The museum presents scenes of vivisection with life-size mannequins, photographs of haggard prisoners, and replicas of the bombs that carried the pathogens of infectious diseases and exploded in isolated areas such as Anda, one hundred kilometers from Pingfang, where prisoner-guinea pigs were tied to posts.

The doctors observed the development of infection in victims whom they had injected with typhoid, dysentery, tetanus, or tuberculosis pathogens, and proceeded with dissection (or more precisely, vivisection) while the victims were still alive. The Japanese called these human guinea pigs *maruta*, which means "logs." The expression has its origin in a gloomy pleasantry: having told the local inhabitants of Pingfang that they were building a sawmill, one member of Unit 731 remarked, as an aside, "and the men are its logs." The incineration of the victims, practically empty of internal organs, was a rapid process, according to a former staff member quoted by Hal Gold in his book *Unit 731: Testimony.*

The history of Unit 731 is one of the more somber pages in the story of Japanese expansionism, and today it is still one of the most obscure. Tokyo has never shed any light on this sinister enterprise. The story owes its research to Japanese and American historians, and to evidence produced by the Chinese—evidence supported by members of Unit 731 who, having regrets in the evening of their lives, described the atrocities committed at Pingfang. In 1982, the Japanese Minister of Health acknowledged that Unit 731 existed, but not the reality of the experiments, stating that the proof was insufficient.

Tokyo has finally admitted to certain crimes committed by the Imperial Army (the massacre of 300,000 noncombatants at Nanking and the "comfort girls" who were forced to prostitute themselves to Japanese soldiers), but Unit 731 remains unmentionable. Yet stonewalling by the

Japanese is not the sole cause. Concerned about keeping the results of the sinister experiments away from the Soviets, the United States actually began the conspiracy of silence; none of the organizers of Unit 731 were investigated by the occupation forces, and the Military Tribunal of Tokyo ignored them even while the Tribunal at Nuremberg condemned their German counterparts as war criminals.

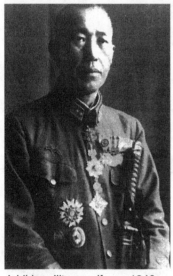
Ishii in military uniform, 1946

Unit 731 shares a sorry distinction with the Nazi doctors; rarely have men gone so far in the systematic negation of others, reducing lives to nothing more than meat for the scalpel. This barbarism can be explained by the attention Japan paid to military hygiene and by the personality of the general commander of Unit 731, the doctor Shiro Ishii, who planned the horror.

Tokyo was quickly persuaded that physical health was worth as much as the force of arms when carrying out a battle. At the beginning of the 20th Century, Japan was the most advanced country in the world in the field of military hygiene. There were Japanese researchers who discovered the causes of beriberi and dysentery. Earning a degree in bacteriology at the Imperial University at Tokyo, Shiro Ishii went on to turn sickness, the "silent enemies" of armies, into "silent allies," according to the expression of Hal Gold. After a journey to Europe, where he studied the chemical weapons used in WWI, he persuaded his superiors of the need for Japan to give itself a bacteriological arsenal, despite Tokyo having signed the Geneva Convention of 1925 banning the use of chemical weapons.

In 1932, when Japan waged the war in China that would lead to Peal Harbor, Ishii took charge of a "research laboratory for the prevention of epidemics" which actually studied biological weapons. Japan felt menaced by the Soviets, who were numerically superior, and so Ishii installed himself next to Harbin, not far from the Soviet border. First at Beiyinhe, a gigantic laboratory-bunker was built that could receive 600 prisoner-guinea pigs. In 1936, after a guinea pig uprising and escape took place and the secrecy of the fortress was compromised, the unit was installed at Pingfang, where it pursued experiments on a larger scale and a practically unlimited budget.

These experiments could be kept secret up to a certain point. The "kanpeitai," or military police, fed the researchers with human guinea pigs. The unit also employed civilian doctors, and it maintained tight relations with hospitals in Japan, where the results of experiments were sent. "The Japanese medical world knew perfectly well how these results had been obtained," estimates Keiichi Tsuneishi, a historian of science and an expert on the history of Unit 731. There was continuous air traffic between Pingfang and Tokyo. Jars of specimens (organs and limbs) arrived from China and were studied at the Army School of Military Health, while tens of thousands of rats left Japan to serve as agents of contamination. Many "settings-free" of rats took place in China after 1937.

Two days before the capitulation of Japan, on August 15, 1945, Unit 731 was shut down as Soviet troops advanced toward Harbin. In order to erase all traces of the activities conducted, the installations were dynamited. "We heard a series of explosions, then some Japanese wearing striped uniforms tore off on foot, heading in the direction of Harbin," Fang Zhen Yu remembers today. Before this, the last 400 prisoners were executed by injections of prussic acid and then incinerated.

Ishii returned to Tokyo by plane, carrying reports and films of the experiments with him. He remained in hiding until one of his "lieutenants," Ryoichi Naito, had obtained immunity for Ishii and all the members of his unit from the U.S. authorities in exchange for the information in his possession. Only twelve members of the unit were put on trial by the Soviets at Khobarovsk in 1949, a trial the U.S. described as "propaganda."

Not only were the members of Unit 731 not prosecuted (Ishii died in his bed in 1959), but they even received pensions, probably from the U.S. Army. Certain ones among them went on to brilliant careers. Naito, Ishii's right hand man who took charge of the unit after 1942, and Hideo Futagi, head of the vivisection team, founded Midori Juji in 1951, a pharmaceutical firm that made a fortune supplying blood to the U.S. Armed Forces in Korea and which has, since 1995, been the center of a scandal involving the infection of hemophiliacs with the AIDS virus. Hideo Tanaka, chief of the plague research team, became President of the Medical College at Osaka. Others climbed through the ranks of the public health care system. In 1994 a list was published in Japan naming 2000 former members of Unit 731.

The Japanese public didn't know of the unit's existence for a long time. Was this the case with Emperor Hirohito? The charter of the unit carried the imperial seal and, according to historian Tsuneishi, the emperor was probably aware of its activities, especially considering the involvement of Princes Mikasa and Takeda, who visited the complex at Pingfang. It was only in 1981, with the publication of the book *Unit 731* by Seiji Morimura

(Rocher editions), that the general public became aware of the sinister activities carried out by Ishii and his team.

On the 50th anniversary of the Japanese surrender, a movement that the veil should be lifted began in the archipelago. In 1993-94 a traveling exposition about Unit 731, which was viewed by 200,000 people, encouraged the testimony of those who had participated in the atrocities. Writes Keichi Tsuneishi in his latest work, *Crimes Organized by Doctors*, "The lamp of truth will not shine until the world of Japanese medicine agrees to recognize the crimes in which it participated and until Washington admits that it covered them up for reasons of high politics."

The Nuremberg Code of Ethics in Medical Research (1948)

1. The voluntary consent of the human subject is absolutely essential.

This means that the person involved should have legal capacity to give consent; should be so situated as to be able to exercise free power of choice, without the intervention of any element of force, fraud, deceit, duress, overreaching, or other ulterior form of restraint or coercion; and should have sufficient knowledge and comprehension of the elements of the subject matter involved as to enable him to make an understanding and enlightened decision. The latter element requires that before the acceptance of an affirmative decision by the experimental subject there should be made known to him the nature, duration, and purpose of the experiment the method and means by which it is to be conducted; all inconveniences and hazards reasonably to be expected; and the effects upon his health or person which may possibly come from his participation in the experiment.

The duty and responsibility for ascertaining the quality of the consent rests upon each individual who initiates, directs or engages in the experiment. It is a personal duty and responsibility which may not be delegated to another with impunity.

2. The experiment should be such as to yield fruitful results for the good of society, unprocurable by other methods or means of study, and not random and unnecessary in nature.

3. The experiment should be so designed and based on the results of animal experimentation and a knowledge of the

natural history of the disease or other problem under study that the anticipated results will justify the performance of the experiment.

4. The experiment should be so conducted as to avoid all unnecessary physical and mental suffering and injury.

5. No experiment should be conducted where there is an *a priori* reason to believe that death or disabling injury will occur; except, perhaps, where the experimental physicians also serve as subjects.

6. The degree of risk to be taken should never exceed that determined by the humanitarian importance of the problem to be solved by the experiment.

7. Proper preparations should be made and adequate facilities provided to protect the experimental subject against even remote possibilities of injury, disability, or death.

8. The experiment should be conducted only by scientifically qualified persons. The highest degree of skill and care should be required through all stages of the experiment of those who conduct or engage in the experiment.

9. During the course of the experiment the human subject should be at liberty to bring the experiment to an end if he has reached the physical or mental state where continuation of the experiment seems to him to be impossible.

10. During the course of the experiment the scientist in charge must be prepared to terminate the experiment at any stage if he has probable cause to believe, in the exercise of the good faith, superior skill, and careful judgment required of him, that a continuation of the experiment is likely to result in injury, disability, or death to the experimental subject.

Why is there a Nuremberg Code?

BY ROBERT HELMS

In 1943, the Nazi anatomists Hermann Voss and Robert Herrlinger performed experiments on Polish resistance fighters at the Gestapo execution site of Posen, occupied Poland. In one example, eight healthy men, ages 18 to 48, were beheaded and made "available" to the anatomists "for blood tests and laparotomy (abdominal dissection) forty to eighty seconds after death." The anatomists were standing beside the guillotine. Herrlinger called the split neck an operating area and described the procedure as follows: "The arterial blood was taken first, from the still-pulsating carotids. Sometimes, however, because of immediate evacuation of chyme (partially digested food) from the esophagus, an accurate examination of the carotid blood became impossible... During the pipetting of the carotid blood, the abdominal cavity was opened, the spleen removed as carefully as possible... a blood sample was taken (from the spleen) on an average of 120-180 seconds post mortem." (See *Cleansing the Fatherland: Nazi Medicine and Racial Hygiene* by Gotz Aly et al., Johns Hopkins, 1994)

For forty years, the US government conducted a syphilis study that actively prevented African-American men from receiving medical treatment for the disease. The subjects were told they were receiving "free medical treatment," not that they were part of a study. An African-American nurse was employed to bridge the cultural gap between the subjects and the researchers. Many of the guinea pigs died of the affliction, while others went blind or insane. An unknown number of women contracted syphilis from the unknowing subjects and congenitally passed the disease on to their children. After the study became a public scandal in 1972, the government admitted that "Nothing learned [from the study] will prevent, find, or cure a single case" of syphilis. Not one person was prosecuted for their part in the study. (See *Bad Blood; The Tuskegee Syphilis Experiment* (2nd ed.) by James H. Jones, Free Press, 1993.)

Dr. Josef Mengele performed bizarre experiments on twins in the concentration camp at Auchwitz. Many of these involved interchanging the blood supplies of different pairs of twins. A witness named Vera Alexander remembered one such experiment:

> One day Mengele brought chocolate and special clothes. The next day, SS men came and brought two children away. They were two of my pets, Tito and Nino. One of them was a hunchback. Two or three days later, the SS men brought them back in a terrible state. They had been cut. The hunchback was sewn to the other child, back to back, their wrists back to back too. There was a terrible smell of gangrene. The cuts were dirty and the children cried every night.

(See Mengele: The Complete Story by G. Posner and J. Ware, McGraw Hill, 1986).

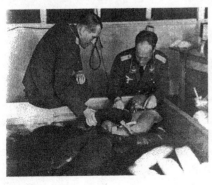

A freezing experiment at the Dachau concentration camp. Two doctors, E. Holzlohner (left) and Sigmund Rascher (right) observe a political prisoner immersed in ice water. (Trial exhibit -Office Chief of Counsel for War Crimes, Nuremberg)

The Skeletons in Ben Franklin's Closet
BY ALISON LEWIS

Benjamin Franklin (1706-1790) is best known for being one of the founding fathers of the United States, acting as elder statesman at the Constitutional Convention and helping to draft the Declaration of Independence. He's also known for exercising freedom of the press to the hilt, and as the brains behind one of the most successful 'zines of all time, Poor Richard's Almanack —you know, where the "A Penny Saved is a Penny Earned" stuff comes from. But what a lot of Americans don't know is that good old Ben actually lived in London from 1757 to 1775, where he served as a representative of the American colonies to the British Parliament. While he was there, he lived with Mrs. Margaret Stevenson, a widow who rented him the upper rooms of her house. Mrs. Stevenson and her daughter, Polly, became something of a second family to Franklin.

Because of the historic significance of the house they lived in, located at No. 36 Craven Street, a group of American and English Franklinophiles purchased the house for renovation. A grisly discovery was made in 1998 when workmen began digging in the basement. Bones. Lots of bones. Lots and lots of bones, all dating from the time period of Franklin's stay in the house. Could our beloved founding father have been involved with some sort of unsavory crime?

Researchers suspect that the bones are actually the products of an anatomy school that met for a time in back of the house. In 1772, Polly Stevenson had married a young physician, William Hewson, and he lived with the family (and Franklin) for two years. Scientists examining the bones say that due to evidence of sawing and drilling characteristic of medical tools of the day they look like they came from the dissection table. Marcia Balisciano, director of the Craven Street House, informed *GPZ* editor Bob Helms and myself on a recent visit that animal bones showing the same sawing and drilling had also been recovered from the garden in front of the house. Hewson was a respected physician, but dissection of human bodies was prohibited at the time his anatomy school operated. The bodies were probably obtained illegally from grave robbers and may have been surreptitiously delivered to the back of the house through a pub on the side street. When the medical students were through practicing their arcane arts, the dissected bodies were secretly buried in the backyard. Years later, the owners built an extension to the house, and the former backyard became the floor of the basement. Hewson unfortunately fell victim to his own experiments: he died of septicemia in 1774, after cutting himself during a dissection. Researchers speculate that Franklin probably knew what was going on in the anatomy school, but that it was unlikely he participated. His scientific interests ran more to physics and natural science than to anatomy and medicine.

Alexis St. Martin (1794-1880): The Intrepid Guinea Pig of the Great Lakes

BY ROBERT HELMS

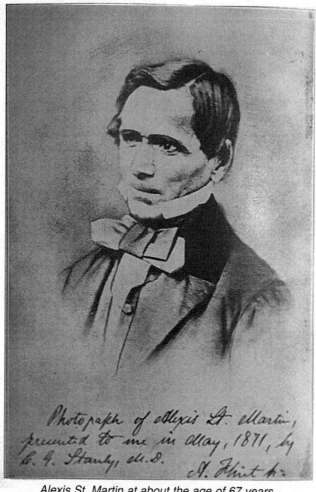

Alexis St. Martin at about the age of 67 years.

Alexis Bidagan dit St. Martin was born on April 18, 1794 in Berthier, Canada, a village north of Montreal. The word *dit* means "called:" he went by St. Martin all his life, but his formal surname was Bidagan. His first name is pronounced "Alexie," as the final "s" is silent. He was a third generation Canadian, his grandfather having come from Bayonne, France. He was the son of Joseph Pierre Bidagan and Marie Des Agnes Angelique Guibeau. This is all that is known of his life before the thunderous sound of a gunshot blasted him into lasting fame.

In 1822 Alexis was a 28 years old voyageur for the American Fur Company at Mackinac Island (sometimes called Machillimackinac), which lies just off the top of the "mitten" of Michigan in Lake Huron. Voyageurs were travelling canoe-men and porters who paddled the big cargo canoes, carrying both the vessel and its cargo along the banks when a waterfall or rapids got in the way. They went in teams, had their own songs and legends, and faced their own special dangers. On the morning of June 6 St. Martin was standing in the company store near someone holding a shotgun loaded for ducks. According to an eye-witness, the muzzle was "not over three feet from him—I think not more than two." At any rate, it accidentally fired, sending the entire charge into the side of St. Martin's chest. Wadding and pieces of cloth entered the wound along with the tiny lead pellets. As he fell to the floor with his shirt on fire, all present believed Alexis was as good as dead. It turned out this was only the start of a long and famous North American guinea pigging adventure.

At the time Mackinac Island was home to a U.S. Army fort and was always filled with Indians and travelers trading their wares or stopping off on their way to somewhere else. The Army surgeon, Dr. William Beaumont, was by all accounts as alert, dedicated and talented as they come. A few minutes after the mishap, Beaumont made his way through the gathering crowd and quickly cleaned and dressed the wound. The doctor then removed the cloth and wadding, trimmed off the ragged edges of the wound, and stanched the bleeding. A dozen years later, Beaumont described first coming upon the famous injury as follows:

> The wound was received just under the left breast, and supposed, at the time, to have been mortal. A large portion of the side was blown off, the ribs fractured and openings made into the cavities of the chest and abdomen, through which protruded portions of the lungs and stomach, much lacerated and burnt, exhibiting altogether an appalling and hopeless case. The diaphragm was lacerated and a perforation made directly into the cavity of the stomach, through which breakfast food was escaping.

The physician remarked to someone assisting him that "the man cannot live thirty-six hours; I will come and see him by and by." To everyone's surprise, however, St. Martin pulled through and began a slow recovery. For 17 days he was sustained by means of nutritious enemas, as all of the food he ate passed out through the wound. Soon afterwards his bowels regained activity, and by the fourth week our young fur trader was eating heartily, digesting normally and crapping like a champ.

For some reason Beaumont gave St. Martin's age as 18 years, and the error was not corrected until the Canadian Physiological Society marked his grave in 1962. Often referring to his patient as a "lad," the doctor was actually just nine years his senior. It is possible that Alexis falsified his age in his dealings with Beaumont, or that the wounded man was never actually asked and someone else stated his age. At any rate, we can be sure that the two men weren't soul mates, being separated by opposite personalities and other accidents of birth. Although both came from rural obscurity, Beaumont was a man of New England Puritan stock who advanced himself to wealth and fame through his thrift and work ethic. Our famous patient-cum-guinea pig was a French-speaking Catholic who spent his money as it came to him, preferred wine over work, and longed to be back on his farm with his family and away from the strange world of science. It was at this stage that Beaumont and St. Martin began raising the eyebrows of history.

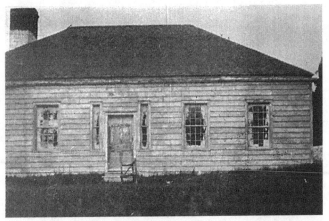

The one-story frame hospital at the old fort, to which Alexis was removed, and where he lay during his long convalescence.

The dedicated physician tended to the gunshot wound and steadily nursed his patient back to health. He achieved success at the point when the man's digestive system was functioning normally and his general state of health was good. Dr. Beaumont wrote of the wound's stabilization in the fifth week as follows:

> By the adhesion of the sides of the protruded portion of the stomach to the *pleura costalis* and the external wound, a free exit was afforded to its contents, and thereby effusion into the abdominal cavity prevented... The stomach became more firmly attached to the pleura and intercostals by its external coat, but showed not the least disposition to close its

orifice by granulations, which terminated as if at a natural boundary, and left the perforation resembling, in all but a sphincter, a natural anus with a slight prolapsus.

What he's saying here is that the hole in the stomach had attached itself to the hole in the side of St. Martin's body, and it just stayed that way. The term for this is a permanent gastric fistula. It was good, he noted, because it kept food from spilling into the body cavity where it didn't belong. He invokes nature as the cause of the fistula that would render his patient a medical circus geek for the rest of his days. "The perforation," he added, "was about the size of a shilling piece... and the food and drinks continually exuded, unless prevented by a plug, compress, and bandage."

It was not all smooth sailing, of course. In the fourth month Beaumont was still removing pieces of gun wadding and shot from abscesses around the wound. The doctor's journals describe many operations to remove unstable pieces of rib and cartilage from the chest. After about ten months, according to the doctor, his wounds were partially healed but he was still "an object miserable and helpless." Alexis was declared a "common pauper" by the civil authorities of the county, who also decided that since they were neither able nor required to look after him, they would send him home to his birthplace "at a distance of more than fifteen hundred miles" by boat.

Once again Dr. Beaumont stepped in and rescued our hero. Believing that the young fellow would be killed by the long journey home, he sort of adopted St. Martin into his own household, and the recovery continued. With the exception of the aperture in the stomach and side, the injured parts were sound, and one year after the accident he was firmly healed.

In April 1824, almost two years after the shotgun accident, Beaumont promoted Alexis from patient to employee. He worked as a sort of factotum, "performing any kind of labor, from that of a house servant to chopping wood or mowing in the field." During his first five months of duty, the doctor noted Alexis did not have "a day's sickness sufficient to disqualify him from his ordinary duties." St. Martin had no complaints of pain or inconvenience save the hassle of applying the compresses over the hole. Whenever he took off the dressing his last meal would spill out, so he had to keep the compress on while he was cleaning up around the doctor's house or tending to the cordwood. So began the one-way scientific love affair between a man and the hole in his patient's stomach. In an 1825 article Beaumont published in The American Medical Recorder, he closes on an optimistic note:

> This case affords a most excellent opportunity of experimenting upon the gastric fluids, and the process of digestion. It would give no pain, nor cause the least uneasiness, to extract a gill of fluid every two or three days, for it frequently flows out spontaneously in considerable quantities; and one might introduce various digestible substances into the stomach, and easily examine them during the whole process of digestion. I may, therefor, be able hereafter to give some interesting experiments on these subjects.

Observe here that Beaumont the scientist took over as Beaumont the doctor stepped out of St. Martin's life. The positive note at the end of that first interesting tale should have been about planning another operation to close up the hole and separate the stomach from the body wall.

This would have restored the patient to his normal state and made him ready to go on his merry way, like any healed patient. William Beaumont never closed the hole, nor did he explain why he chose not to; this point entered public debate in 1834 when Beaumont asked for government money to support his research. The debate gained further importance in the Darnes-Davis murder case of 1840, when it was used to shift the blame of a death from the batterer to the surgeon who attempted to save the victim's life.

That trial deserves brief description: In 1840, when Beaumont was practicing in St. Louis, a politician met a newspaper editor on the street and bashed in the latter's skull with an iron cane because of his treatment in the paper's editorials. Beaumont was one of several surgeons who treated the editor. He decided to use a kind of hole-saw called a trephine to relieve pressure on the brain through a circular hole in the patient's skull. The lawyer for the politician brought up the case of Alexis St. Martin as an example of Beaumont's scientific interests taking precedence over the welfare of a patient. The lawyer declared that "it was upon the same principle of curiosity which kept the hole open in the man's stomach that he bored a hole in the editor's head to see what was going on there!" On this premise the lawyer put the question to the jury: Did the editor die from his wounds or from the treatment of his doctors? The defendant walked away with a $500 fine, and Beaumont's reputation suffered a blow.

However, Beaumont did gain from not closing St. Martin's wound. The doctor never questioned his own ethics, but simply raved for the rest of his life about the wonders he and other researchers would find inside St. Martin's magic hole. As a leading physiologist, Beaumont gained enormous prestige and a permanent place in the history of human research off St. Martin. To this day wax figures of the two are displayed at Fort Mackinac, and Beaumont's writings are still on the shelves of university libraries throughout the world. It would be difficult to accept that the physician did not actively manipulate the situation to his own benefit. Beaumont wasn't incompetent, like some mechanic who could rebuild an engine but couldn't change a flat tire. Beaumont allowed his curiosity to take precedent over the well-being of his patient, kind of like a heart surgeon leaving a chest open to watch the repaired organ function for 60 years. This patient was denied the most obvious part of any treatment—closure. Beaumont's subsequent use of St. Martin as an experimental subject shows the surgeon to be both exploitive and unethical.

Beaumont's modern biographer, Reginald Horsman, explains the frontier doctor's attitude was average for his times:

> ...There were no concerned thoughts about the psychological effects of a permanent gastric fistula on this Canadian voyageur, no concerns about the mental effects of repeated tampering with his normal process of digestion, nor even any particular concern about the destitute condition of his family... Beaumont's attitude toward St. Martin was probably as good as most. He had no concern about the ethics of his experiments, but no one else did either. He was not an unkind man, but as a physician he was a man of his age.

The stomach experiments began in May 1825, and the subject traveled with his employer to Fort Niagara, NY; Burlington, VT; and then Plattsburgh, NY. Then the robust Alexis decided he'd exposed his accidental aperture to enough intrusions for one year, and skipped out to make his way home to Berthier. Here he married Marie Joly, and together they had six children: Alexis Jr., Charles, Henriette, Marie, and two whose names are not recorded in any published records. Taking up his old fur trading profession with another firm, he remained in Canada for four years until the diligent Dr. Beaumont tracked him down through St. Martin's former employer, American Fur Company. These agents hired the great guinea pig on Beaumont's behalf and transported him and his family nearly 2,000 miles by boat to Fort Crawford in Prairie du Chien, Wisconsin (in those days an extremely rugged trip). They arrived in August, 1829, and the doctor happily observed that no change had developed in the precious hole during his subject's absence. The St. Martin family remained at Fort Crawford almost for two years and had two of their six children there. The second series of experiments was performed at Fort Crawford under the same arrangement as before, i.e. with Alexis as human guinea pig and general servant for Beaumont.

It was probably at Fort Crawford that an incident occurred between Alexis' brother Etienne and a Charlie Charette, who had been ridiculing "the man with the lid on his stomach." According to an anecdote passed down from a neighbor, Etienne stabbed the tormentor, wounding him "quite severely," and swore that he would "kill the whole brigade" if they didn't lay off his brother. Alexis and his family departed in March, 1831, apparently because of Mrs. St. Martin's "homesickness and discontent." In later years Beaumont reminded his subject of the

> embarrassment and interruption that have occurred heretofore to the prosecution of my experiments upon you on account of having your family with you [at Prairie du Chien]... you know your wife became so discontented and determined to go back

that you were obliged to yield to her and disappoint me.

St. Martin took his wife and four children in an open canoe "via the Mississippi, passing St. Louis, ascending the Ohio to the lakes, and descended the Erie and Ontario and the river St. Lawrence to Montreal, where they arrived in June." On the occasion of this second departure, Beaumont proudly described the method of travel used by Alexis to illustrate the completeness of his recovery and the ease with which he lived with the extra orifice.

In the fall of 1832 Alexis again signed on with

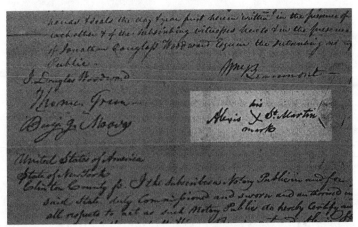

Signature of Alexis St. Martin

Beaumont, and the pair embarked on a third series of experiments in Plattsburgh and Washington DC. In 1833 Beaumont made use of his friendship with Surgeon General Joseph Lovell to have St. Martin enrolled in the US Army, in a Washington detachment of orderlies, as a sergeant. He would receive $12 a month and a few allowances, and his only duty was to make himself available to Dr. Beaumont as an experimental subject. The enlistment records note St. Martin's height was 5'5".

Alexis' responsibilities to the Army were never taken

seriously by anyone. Indeed, he and Beaumont retained their subject/scientist terms of service both before and after St. Martin's enlistment. The first contract was signed on October 16, 1832, for one year at $150 plus food and lodging, with St. Martin agreeing to follow the doctor wherever he might go in the world. The second contract was signed on November 7, 1833, for two years at $400. In each case, Alexis was paid $40 up front. The month of the second contract also saw the last recorded experiment that Beaumont ever performed on the savvy businessman. These contracts, of course, would have been unnecessary between a soldier and his Commanding Officer, but the regular Army pay would never have persuaded a sane person to regularly whore out his fistula. The arrangement was established so Alexis could cover his own travel and food costs while in Beaumont's service.

At any rate, the Doctor was transferred to Jefferson Barracks, Missouri shortly after the second contract was signed. While Beaumont was in DC shopping for scientific books to bring along, he arranged for St. Martin to take a short leave of absence and meet him in Plattsburgh. Beaumont had approached the U.S. Congress for research funding and was arranging for demonstrations in major cities on both sides of the Atlantic, but the Canadian never appeared. The funding and demonstrations of course depended upon St. Martin's presence, so his truancy came at an especially embarrassing moment for the scientist. Yet, no attempt was ever made to capture or impose military discipline upon Alexis, even though he had deserted his military post. Looking back on the event, Beaumont told another scientist that Alexis' return was prevented "partly from the situation of his family and its affairs, but more perhaps from the natural obstinacy of his disposition and unwillingness to submit himself for public experiments..."

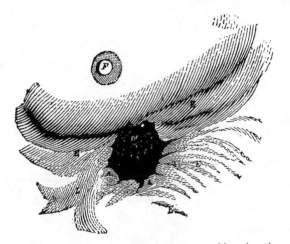

Engraving of the aperature with valve depressed

In 1833 Beaumont published his book *Experiments and Observations on the Gastric Juice and the Physiology of Digestion*. This contains some 240 experiments, all performed on the same famous stomach and earning the Army Surgeon no small prestige. It included diet tables that were used as authoritative texts for almost a century. His work with St. Martin proved that digestion was a chemical process, ending a debate on this matter that dated from the earliest annals of medicine. In 1835 Beaumont was appointed Medical Officer of the St. Louis Arsenal. Resigning his commission in 1840, he lived on a farm outside the city and remained active in the medical societies of the region. He remained there until his death in 1853. Many of Beaumont's letters survive, and these tell of his unceasing and always disappointed efforts to re-hire Alexis as his experimental subject. The letters also provide useful details of Alexis' life and whereabouts.

Another interesting point is how historians have chosen to quote only particular letters by St. Martin. Certain elements of St. Martin's letters, like the following dated May 24, 1843 and quoted by Meyer, were excluded from historical accounts: "...I have not forgot you. I have had some sickness in my family, and lost two of my children [including Alexis Jr.], and was unwell myself for the best part of a year." This sort of revelation shows the guinea pig was not just some ungrateful servant, but a person.

One wouldn't know that from the following letter. In 1939 Arno B. Luckhardt, library curator at the University of Chicago, wrote a summary about the donation of Beaumont's papers to his collection. One letter from St. Martin to the doctor is dated December 19, 1834. By that time Alexis has settled his family on a small farm fifteen miles southwest of Berthier, at a place called La Chalaupe. All of the agents sent by Beaumont reported that the family was very poor, and in one letter that all of them were "destitute of clothing." Just as interesting as the letter's contents are the curator's introduction and footnote to it. Alexis was illiterate, which wasn't unusual at the time, and had someone else (probably the parish priest) write replies to the doctor's letters. The curator begins: "The translated text of this letter is representative of many others written by the surly, irresponsible, pecunious, ungrateful ward and human guinea pig to his solicitous, merciful, and generous benefactor reads as follows:

Dear Doctor:

I am surprised and mortified (at the same time) not to have received any answer to my letters, except by personal communication of William Morrison. However, I should have much desired to join you. I have even started to go there and had gotten as far as St. John, but illness caused me to go back. I was throwing up blood. I decided to write to you from St. John to let you know. I should have yielded to your desire expressed to me by Mr. Morrison if it had not been that I fell ill, as I just told you. In case you wish to have me with you again I should be very glad to join you with my family and in sending me some money, in settling my account you will see some money is due me. I should wish to have seven or eight Louis to take care of my family and at your request I should be ready to go, Sir, I shall wait for your answer with diligence. As I am thinking of cultivating my land myself, if I do not go with you, I should wish to have an answer from you about it. For if I began to cultivate my land I could not go. My wife and family join me to send you our regards (and also your wife), and I desire much to see you. And we end by wishing you good health and all sorts of prosperity in calling myself

Your Affectionate Servant,
Alexis St. Martin

After the letter, the curator chimes in again:

Prof. Henri David of the University of Chicago kindly prepared this literal translation from the original "French." [...] The content of the letter prompts the reflection that in enduring fame, "Extremes Meet!" In this instance, Alexis St. Martin will continue to engage the attention of posterity because of the genius of William Beaumont.

Luckhardt's remarks are pregnant with problems, the least of which is that a swaggering opinion has no right place in an article describing the acquisitions of a university archive. But it stands as a fine example of a person of relative privilege with a compulsion to abuse working people, even where no opinion is asked—not a far cry from Beaumont. It also gives an insight as to how human research subjects have been historically viewed: as servants of their learned manipulators who should be grateful to be in such distinguished company and who are human only in the mechanical sense. Luckhardt's editors let his highbrow cretinism remain.

However, even Jesse Meyer's biography has been reigned in a bit for its elaborate discussion of the guinea pig hero. The original 1912 edition has become rare and expensive, but in 1981 its publisher released a special reprint edition under an amended title. Both of the two known images of Alexis at the time of publication were included in the original edition, but one was omitted in the reprint while pictures of upper-class persons and bit-players were included for the first time.

From St. Martin's departure from Washington in 1833 until Beaumont's death in 1853, the doctor tried desperately to persuade his subject to resume experiments. However, no agreement was ever reached, and the two men never saw each other again. The intermediaries sent by Beaumont included his son Israel, but none were able to lure him to St. Louis. The main sticking point was that Alexis would not relocate without his family, and he insisted that Beaumont find them lodging as well as employment. While he was living in Canada he had to work his fields according to the iron law of seasons that grips every farmer. The intermediaries did, however, observe his "wretched" poverty and his inclination to drink. His wife, who appears to have been a person of strong personality, insisted that she and the little ones come along for fear that they would starve without Alexis. On June 26, 1836, Alexis wrote Dr. Beaumont:

> My wife is not willing for me to go, for she thinks that I can do a great deal better to stay at home, for on my farm she thinks there will be a great deal more profit for me ... I hope you won't be angry with me, for I can do better at home. I am much obliged

to you for what you have done, and if it was in my power, I should do all I could for you with pleasure.

In one attempt to recruit the great lab rat back into service, Dr. Beaumont asked fur trader William Morrison to visit St. Martin, "if you can endure the disagreeable condescension of seeing Alexis..." In a letter to his cousin Samuel Beaumont, the surgeon asked his cousin to bring Alexis to him "dead or alive, with or without his live stock." These remarks and many others illustrate the scientist's attitude toward his experimental subject. In an 1847 letter to his son, the doctor carefully instructs him not to become an equal to an illiterate man of the lower class:

> ...You will take him in charge as a private servant in traveling. Keep him in his place, and strictly control his time and services. Allow no undue familiarity, or suffer him to take the slightest advantage of your age and inexperience ... [If he should] give you much trouble ... discharge him at once ... and proceed without him.

There are two reports of other medical groups attempting to obtain the services of St. Martin while Beaumont was still living, but neither was successful. In 1837 a group of physicians promoting vegetarianism sought to bring St. Martin to Boston in the hopes of disproving Beaumont's claim that meat was easier to digest than veggies. In 1840 the Medical Society of London raised 300-400 British Pounds to seduce Alexis across the Atlantic to show them the hole. These attempts worried Beaumont, so he sweetened his offers for St. Martin's services. But St. Martin was loyal to the man who saved his life; it was only after Beaumont's death that he took his wares elsewhere. Toward the end of his life Dr. Beaumont regretted his refusal to include St. Martin's family in the deal. Letters to friends reveal that he looked back on the whole affair of St. Martin's services as one that could have been resolved with a decisive investment of money. Beaumont died in April 1853 from injuries suffered from a fall on ice-covered steps earlier that March.

From April through July of 1856, a new and sadder chapter in Alexis' life occurred under the influence of a true charlatan named Dr. Bunting. As this episode unfolds we can see that St. Martin may have regretted the passing of his former employer. The tour covered more than ten cities in the eastern U.S. and Canada, including Boston, Cincinnati, Columbus, Detroit, Louisville, Montreal, New York, Philadelphia, St. Louis, and Toronto. Edward Bensley, a medical historian whose research has given new life to this intrepid human guinea pig, concludes that the pair must have stopped at many other sites as well. The medical men in all but one of the documented cities observed that Bunting was a fake and the 62-year old man with the perforated chest was a sorry drunk. The considerable press exposure drew the attention of the circus master P. T. Barnum, but Alexis never found himself under the big top.

Bunting was a snake-oil dealer of very ill repute before beginning his enterprise with our hero. In January 1850 he came to Montreal and advertised a cure for stammering and stuttering in a local paper. He used Dr. William Marsden of Quebec City as a reference. This was a rather clumsy move, as Marsden immediately published a disclaimer in a respectable medical journal stating he had never witnessed any such cure, but that he had met Bunting. The charlatan had introduced himself to Marsden as a member of the College of Surgeons of London, but when Marsden checked with the college,

Bunting's claim proved false.

In June 1856, Alexis and this "impostor, swindler, and villain," as the press called Bunting, visited Mrs. Beaumont in St. Louis so Alexis could pay his respects to the widow of his former employer. Alexis, who was described by the doctor's son Israel as "a thin, meager-faced, much bronzed little Frenchman," asked after the other children and wished the whole family well. The bogus medicine man regaled the old lady with stories of how he knew her late husband's publisher and how he would be republishing his works when he and St. Martin extended their tour into Europe.

Another episode that stands apart from this garish tour was St. Martin's examination in Philadelphia under Dr. Francis Gurney Smith. Smith conducted a few more experiments published in the Philadelphia Medical Examiner, but these were generally regarded as less important than Beaumont's experiments. It does, however, seem to be the one occasion where Bunting was able to rub elbows with real scientists through the famous human subject. Dr. Smith reported:

> [On] May 6th, 1856, at 10 a.m., two ounces of dry wheat bread were given to St. Martin, which he masticated deliberately and swallowed. At 12:30 p.m., the contents of the stomach were removed by Dr. Bunting in the presence of a number of medical gentlemen and students, and carefully preserved for immediate analysis.

He also mentioned that "during all the experiments St. Martin maintained his usual good health, was in excellent spirits, and took his food with appetite."

St. Martin was doing fine in the 1850's, and well beyond. Meyer's biography of Beaumont states that in

1870 Alexis and his family were living in Cavendish, Vermont, where he earned his living by "chopping wood by the cord." This is remarkable, as the man was 76 years old, but it could also be an affectionate exaggeration of his health and activity. His four surviving children, though grown and married, were living with him in abject poverty. At the time he frequently corresponded with Israel Beaumont. In 1879 St. Martin returned to Canada, settling in St. Thomas de Joliette, very close to his birthplace. Shortly after the move, he wrote to Israel:

> ...I am beginning to get old, and I have been ill for six years, and I will not hide from you that I am very poor... I am suffering a little from my gastric fistula, and my digestion grows worse than ever... In granting me your charity... you will not be inconvenienced for long, as I am old and sick.

William Osler preserved another late description of our hero in his introduction to the 1929 reprint of Beaumont's book. A certain Judge Baby of the town of Joliette (near Berthier), described St. Martin as follows:

> When I came to know St. Martin it must have been a few years before his death. A lawsuit brought him to my office here in Joliette. I was seized with his interests; he came to my office a good many times, during which visits he spoke to me at great length of his former life, how his wound had been caused, his peregrinations through Europe and the United States, etc. He showed me his wound. He complained bitterly of some doctors who had awfully misused him, and had kind words for others. He had made considerable money during his tours, but he had expended and thrown it all away in a frolic-

some way, especially in the old country. When I came across him he was rather poor, living on a small, scanty farm in St. Thomas, and very much addicted to drink, almost a drunkard one might say. He was a tall, lean man, with a very dark complexion, and appeared to me then of a morose disposition.

The judge's report is interesting because it describes Alexis as "tall" and has him remembering trips to Europe. The Army record of his height was quoted by Osler as 5'5, but the rural poor in those days were often much shorter. Apparently he was taller than average. There were at least two known attempts to get the punctured geezer to Europe, as described above, but there is no sure evidence from the other side of the Atlantic of any such trips— although in 1834 a small bottle of Alexis' gastric juices did make the trip. Dr. Beaumont had sent a sample to the renowned chemist Benjamin Silliman in Sweden. He was later disappointed to learn that because of the summer heat and the five-month journey overseas, Silliman declined to analyze the specimen since he could not be sure it still retained the properties of fresh gastric juice.

Alexis St. Martin died at St. Thomas de Joliette, Quebec on June 24, 1880, and was buried in the cemetery of that parish on June 28. A Catholic funeral mass was held by a Reverend Chicoine. The body was in such an advanced state of decomposition that it could not be brought into the church, so it remained outside during the service. Dr. William Osler had wanted the three-holed gut to reside permanently in the Army Medical Museum in Washington, but the family had refused the "most pressing" requests from the medical profession for any autopsy or purchase of the famous stomach. Relatives even kept Alexis' body at home longer than usual during a hotspell in the hopes that the body would decompose to be as little use as possible to science. The family also dug his grave 8 feet deep rather than 6 to prevent "resurrectionists" in the employ of doctors from robbing the grave. Marie St. Martin lived for several years after her husband's death.

Some eighty years after the great guinea pig passed away, members of a fine Canadian group decided that the man whose humble stomach helped us learn so much should be acknowledged for his contributions. With a level of gratitude that is all too rare among medical professionals, they declared:

> In recalling the memory of Alexis St. Martin the Canadian Physiological Society wished to encompass all the passive collaborators of science, all the patients who without prospect of immediate benefit contribute nonetheless to the growth and development of science. But most of all the society wishes to pay homage to Alexis, the uneducated man who consented to make the long trips of several months' duration in the great canoes, to be separated from his family for years on end, and to endure who knows how many other forgotten discomforts, in order to be of service to that pioneer of physiology William Beaumont.

They then formed a committee that located the gravesite, looked up his descendants and gave St. Martin a plaque in a proper ceremony. The bronze plaque is engraved in both French and English, with a cross in the center. The English, which reads a little less graciously than the French, says:

In Memory of Alexis Bidagan dit St. Martin

Born April 18, 1794 at Berthier
Died June 24, 1880 at St. Thomas

Buried June 28, 1880 in an unmarked grave close by this tablet. Grievously injured by the accidental discharge of a shotgun on June 6, 1822 at Machillimackinac, Michigan, he made a miraculous recovery under the care of Dr. William Beaumont, Surgeon in the United States Army. After his wounds had healed, he was left with an opening into the stomach and became the subject of Dr. Beaumont's pioneering work on the physiology of the stomach. Through his affliction he served all humanity. Erected by the Canadian Physiological Society, June 1962.

The human guinea pigs of today can proudly look

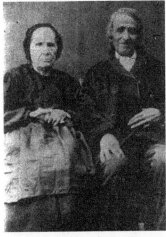 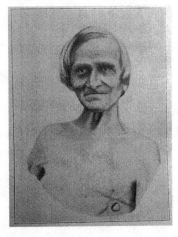

Alexis St. Martin and his wife Marie in old age (courtesy of Tamara Sears)

Alexis St. Martin at the age of 81 years

back to the strong, shrewd, and intrepid St. Martin. He used his experience in commerce to get the most for his services to Beaumont, but did not let his life be drained of all its joys for the progress of science or the glory of one man. Like Alexis St. Martin, we who sacrifice our health and comfort, travel far from our homes and families for uncertain payment, and lay down our flesh for the benefit of humanity should cherish the memory of this noble pioneer. Let him be called our patron saint, our hero, or our historical poster child, but let us never forget him. The awareness of our own history is an armor that can fend off society's abuse and holds our pride close against our hearts. None are so needy of this armor than we, the wandering lab rats of the modern medical jungle.

For Further reading:
Beaumont, William. *Experiments and Observations on the Gastric Juice and the Physiology of Digestion.* Boston: no pub, 1929. With biographical essay by Sir William Osler.

[Beaumont, William] Joseph Lovell. "A Case of Wounded Stomach." *Medical Recorder 8* (January 1825): 14-19.

Bensley, Edward H. "Alexis St. Martin and Dr. Bunting." *Bulletin of the History of Medicine 44* (March-April 1970): 127-32.

Committee of Commemoration of Alexis Bidagan dit St. Martin of the Canadian Physiological Society. "Alexis St. Martin Commemorated." *Physiologist 6* (1963): 63-65.

Horsman, Reginald. *Frontier Doctor: William Beaumont, America's First Great Medical Scientist.* Columbia and London: University of Missouri Press, 1996.
Luckhardt, Arno B. "The Dr. William Beaumont

Collection of the University of Chicago." *Bulletin of the History of Medicine 5* (May 1939) 535-63.

Meyer, Jesse S., comp. *Life and Letters of Dr. William Beaumont, Including Hitherto Unpublished Data Concerning the Case of Alexis St. Martin,* by Jesse S. Meyer. Introduction by Sir William Osler. St. Louis: C.V. Mosby, 1912.

Meyer, Jesse S., et al. *William Beaumont: A Pioneer American Physiologist.* St. Louis: C.V. Mosby, 1981.

Numbers, Ronald L. "William Beaumont and the Ethics of Human Experimentation." *Journal of the History of Biology 12* (Spring 1979) 113-35.

"The Window in St. Martin's Stomach." *Readers' Digest,* October 1951.

Smith, Francis G. "Experiments Upon Digestion." *Medical Examiner 12* (July & September 1856). 385-94; 513-18.

Widdler, Keith R.: *Reveille Till Taps: Soldier Life at Fort Mackinac 1780-1895.* (1972)

Williams, Meade C. *Early Mackinac: A Sketch.* (1987)

Osborn, Chase. "Beaumont—Citizen." *Physician and Surgeon 22* (December 1900) 588-91.

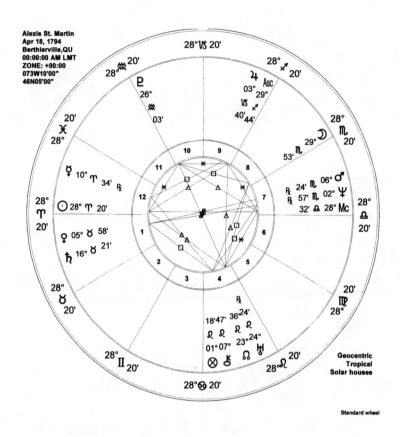

Alexis St. Martin
Apr 18, 1794
Berthierville,QU
00:00:00 AM LMT
ZONE: +00:00
073W10'00"
46N05'00"

Geocentric
Tropical
Solar houses

Standard wheel

The above is a version of the natal astrology chart for the famous human guinea pig, Alexis St. Martin. The close conjunction between his Mars and Neptune in Scorpio may indicate his alcoholism; an "afflicted" Neptune is often seen in cases of addiction. The close trine between his Jupiter in Capricorn and his Venus in Taurus, however, must have softened his personality somewhat and given him some creative abilities, perhaps in the practical realm of crafts. But of particular note here are some of the deeper, "karmic" influences which might reflect Mr. St. Martin's strange fate. First of all, his "part of fortune" in the chart (circle with X through it) is at 1 degree of Leo, conjunct with an orb of 6 degrees the asteroid Chiron. Chiron is known as "the wounded healer" and thus is a most apropos metaphor for Mr. St. Martin; his unfortunate wounding accident created a laboratory where human physiology could be studied in a way never before possible, and the knowledge gained there surely benefited and helped to heal other sufferers. Mr. St. Martin, although he could be seen as doubly victimized by his condition, did however receive monetary gain as a result of it, an occurrence often associated with the part of fortune. Likewise, the North Node (shaped like a horseshoe) is conjunct within 1 degree to the planet Uranus. The North Node is karmic, showing where one is heading in this life, and Uranus is often associated with the unusual or the unexpected. The unusual incident of Mr. St. Martin's wounding definitely altered the course of his life in unexpected ways, and even gained him a footnote in medical history.

NOTE: *Normally, three elements are necessary for erecting an accurate birth chart: date of birth, place of birth, and time of birth. Since no data is available concerning Mr. St. Martin's time of birth. I have erected a solar chart, i.e. one that places the Sun on the ascendant. Because this method has been used, the house placements of the planets and the degree and sign of the fast-moving Moon are likely not accurate and so are not considered. Berthierville is the modern name for Berthier, Quebec.*

ALISON M. LEWIS

Sorry I'm so Late, But the Phone Kept Ringing...

BY ROBERT HELMS

Since the release of *Guinea Pig Zero* #5, the past nine months have been another big adventure, which kept me from getting to the next issue. The principle distraction has been all the media attention. Every time some journalist wants to do a story, it takes all kinds of time. First comes the phone tag, then the first long chat, then the interview, and then they finally leave me alone and take it from there. Sometimes they want a short piece, which requires less time, and sometimes they want to do a long, involved piece, which takes forever. Sometimes a story or TV segment comes from this work, and sometimes it all ends up on the cutting room floor. In other words, for every time the media runs a mention, a quote, a segment, or a feature story on me and my strange little zine, it means a good many hours of lost time. I almost never get paid for any of this, and when I do it's for consulting, not for being written about.

Having said that, I'll mention the more conspicuous media moments where I surfaced and spouted pearls of wisdom into the listening universe. Since January there has been *ABC News 20/20*, *People Magazine*, *The Associated Press*, several long radio interviews for stations all over the U.S. and Canada, *TV Globo* from Brazil, and numerous interviews for other magazines, newspapers, zines, and their counterparts in cyberspace. I was even reviewed in naughty old *Genesis Magazine*, and I got four devils—hubba hubba! There's a TV documentary in the works; I've advised on the script of a comedy portraying college-aged guinea pigs; I've spoken to small local gatherings, and professors in a few colleges are now assigning

GPZ to their students. I also spoke to a class at Temple University, and just as I was explaining the guinea pig routines and how I usually get a catheter in the arm before dosing time, a young student in the front row passed out and landed on the classroom floor. For once I didn't know what the hell to say. He came to a few seconds later, saying "last thing I remember was him talking about his veins..." We lab rats sometimes forget how weird and gory our job can seem to outsiders.

All this has gone to my head, of course, but I've spent so much time on the same subject matter that I'm already tired of it. There's only so much a person can say about one area of interest, especially when the talking takes me away from spending time in libraries and doing other drug studies so I can learn new things to say. But I have been doing other studies and painting houses to make my living.*

There has been another footnote on the 1997 libel suit filed against me and *Harper's Magazine* by the Allegheny hospital chain. Allegheny has gone belly-up! Remember how I called Allegheny CEO Sherif Abdelhak "the robber-baron of Pennsylvania hospitals?" Well, just in case you thought I was railing against him for strictly personal reasons, please know that all my prophesies have come to pass. Abdelhak was fired about a week before bankruptcy was filed in June. Since then the court has been trying to sell what's left of the company. An early bid of $465 million (for 8 city hospitals) was withdrawn after a few weeks because so many physicians had packed up and fled, sharply reducing the value of the company. The new bid is for about $100 million less. A week or so later subpoenas were served on Allegheny's former officers and staff attorneys; authorities are wondering why Abdelhak

---

* By the way, there's plenty of room for a new zine entitled *House Painter*.

formed little satellite companies around his 'non-profit' foundation with the sole purpose of buying him mansions. Now the new buyers are asking for a postponement of the sale because they can't get any respectable teams to manage Allegheny's medical college. As I write, the latest development is that all the other Philadelphia hospitals are drawing up emergency plans for the possible sudden closure of some or all of the ruined hospitals. Everyone in town has favorite anecdotes from the collapse, like "It was unbelievable. They were borrowing gauze pads from other hospitals because their suppliers had cut them off and no one would extend them credit!"

The gist of the matter is that *Harper's Magazine*, my sometime co-defendant, would have shared a victory with me if they had simply read the writing on the wall instead of the fearful letterhead of Abdelhak's attorney. Even Dick Sprague, the most powerful lawyer in Philly and the top gun for libel suits in the U.S., cannot defend a guy who has brought eight of the finest hospitals on earth to ruin. *Guinea Pig Zero* stands tall and proud, *Harper's* squirms with shame for having cracked under pressure, the Allegheny empire is on its belly begging for help, and for the time being Abdelhak walks away from the mess with wads of cash in his pockets. As for Allegheny's "hell-hole" research unit that I criticized in *GPZ #2*, (and in so doing started the whole battle), it has been closed down for good, just as I recommended in the first place.

Why do I write this zine? What compels me to obsess about all these larger-than-life issues upon which I can have only the smallest effect? Let me offer a little family folklore tale to illustrate why it's always worth it:

Once upon a time (around 1959) in West Babylon, Long Island, a nice Irish gal named Mary Helms was fixing some lunch while her little boy Bobby was standing in his playpen watching her with wide eyes (that's me). From out in the backyard, under a trellis of grape leaves, her four-year old daughter Denise called out; "Mommy, a man's taking Josh!"

Mary leaned over to peer out the kitchen window. A uniformed dogcatcher was opening the gate of our short chain-link fence and taking our Saint Bernard, Josh by the collar. To Mary's amazement, he then walked the slobber-monster out through the gate and loaded him into the back of his truck. Fortunately, telephones had already been invented. Mary reached over and dialed the number of the Mandra Brothers Gulf Station in the nearby town of Wyandanch, where her husband was busy fixing cars. "Bob!" she gasped, "The dogcatcher's taking Josh! He was in the yard, minding his own business and the guy came in and got him!"

Bob Sr. knew where the dog pound was, so he put down the phone and fired up his 1949 Mercury convertible. He drove toward home along Straight Path, and just as approached Edison Avenue and signaled to turn he spotted the dogcatcher's truck turning down the same road from the opposite direction. Bob Helms followed close on his tail, and there in the rear window of the truck was the noble face of Josh, a prize-winning pedigreed pooch whose good breeding and pleasant demeanor made up for his obvious lack of watch-dogginess.

The dog truck pulled in behind the dog warden's office, and Bob parked his Mercury in the front lot. Marching in the office door, he demanded his dog.

"Er, what kind of dog was it?" the warden inquired.

"He's a Saint Bernard. Let's see him!" Bob said firmly.

"We don't have any Saint Bernards," said the public servant. "Where did you lose this dog?"

"Baloney. I just saw him in the truck, and my wife saw the guy take him out of the yard."

"Look, pal, you can't tell us..." the warden began.

Bob ignored the shifty thief and summoned his faithful hound: "Josh!" "WOOOOF!" came the deep reply.

The lean mechanic reached behind the low office gate and unlatched it. Before the warden could speak he tapped the warden's shoulder, commanded him to "step aside," and calmly opened the steel mesh gate leading to the animal pens. In the roar of some ten or twelve barking mongrels he spotted Josh, tongue lolling, tail wagging, and drool dribbling as usual. The iron cage that held him was just slightly taller than he was. Bob opened the cage and Josh licked his hand and followed him out through the office. "Come to my house again," he assured the sheepish warden, "and I'll break your scrawny back. Understand?" There was no response.

This strange occurrence took a month or so to explain, but after asking around and picking over the grapevine for information, Bob and Mary learned that certain medical laboratories were trying to perfect the art of heart transplantation. Large dogs were being purchased for experimental surgery because their hearts were about the same size as a human's. They were too big to breed like rats or rabbits, so sneaky surgeons bought household hounds from dirty dog-nappers. It seemed clear that the dog warden had wanted to sell our poor pooch down the drainpipe of science for a few dollars. Who knows how many Labradors, Great Danes, and Rotweilers perished under the knife for every slobbering Saint Bernard that was saved?

Enjoy the zine, and don't take any wooden nickels.

The Toxic Theater: Human Experimentation and the Gulf War
BY BETH LAVOIE

The Persian Gulf War will be remembered by most Americans as a victorious electronic orgy that flooded our evening news with video game tactics. After nearly a decade, the memory of our collective conscience has reduced this war to smart bombs, yellow ribbons, and the perfect bad guy. To quote a nameless soldier, "it was like a turkey shoot!" A clean precise war that we won with few memorial walls attached.

Only the war never ended. Behind the wall of a virtual media blackout we continue to bomb; the economic sanctions bring slow death to a generation of Iraqis; and our own Gulf War veterans are still fighting for their lives and the lives of their children.

Gulf War troops faced many threats on the front lines, probably the least of which were the Iraqis. Years after the official conflict, many veterans are struggling with the toxic aftermath of "friendly fire." Unexplained illnesses plague these men and women. The symptoms suggest exposure to depleted uranium (DU) and experimental drugs. The Pentagon denies any and all knowledge, denies the danger of these substances, denies the exposure, and denies the sickness altogether despite documentation stating otherwise. Shrouded in the iron veil of military secrecy, another page in the Pentagon's long history of reckless human experimentation is being written.

Depleted Uranium
The Department of Defense (DOD), in its gleeful search for ever smarter weaponry, developed a depleted uranium tipped missile. DU is essentially nuclear waste. When ura-

nium is mined, the more radioactive uranium is removed and used in nuclear weapons and reactors. The waste product is depleted uranium. DU has a radioactive half-life of 4.5 billion years. Its extreme density (1.6 times as dense as lead) and ability to burn make it attractive for use in weapons.[1] Its armor piercing ability has made it the "penetrator" of choice for knocking out armored vehicles. U.S. Army test data shows that when a DU penetrator impacts a target, between 20 and 70 percent of the round burns, scattering an extremely fine uranium dust in and around the target.

DU poses the greatest danger to human health when it is inhaled, ingested, or it contaminates a wound. According to U.S. military studies and other independent reports, an intake of DU can cause kidney and liver damage, lung and bone cancer, leukemia, birth defects, and immune system damage.[2]

The Pentagon used these penetrators with a vengeance. Throughout Desert Storm combat, 631,000 pounds of DU was released—enough radioactive and toxic waste to poison every American man, woman, and child 100 times over.[3]

The military had this knowledge, yet did not provide training to combat personnel likely to be exposed, nor did they conduct the thorough post-combat environmental cleanups necessary to prevent further contamination and risk to public health. Furthermore, after demolishing Iraq's armed forces, the Army needlessly exposed U.S. troops to DU by allowing them to re-enter, unprotected and uninformed, the theater for "battlefield tours." The soldiers unwittingly struck victory poses, took pictures, and dug for souvenirs around incinerated Iraqis tanks. The war was over, and as they were breathing deep sighs of

---

[1] <u>DU Case Narrative</u>, Dan Fahey, 3rd Edition, Sept. 20, 1998 p. 10.

[2] ibid.

[3] ibid p. ii.

relief they surely inhaled the remnant DU dust coating the refuse and blowing undetected in the sandy desert air.

Experimental Vaccines and Drugs

Ironically, the second blast of friendly fire came in the form of "protection." The U.S. in part supplied Iraq with its chemical/biological arsenal, including the sale of anthrax as late as the spring of 1990 (note: this date is after Iraq gassed the Kurds). Suspecting Iraq might use this arsenal, the U.S. military sought to provide some kind of defense for its troops. The only possibilities were two experimental vaccines for anthrax and botulism, and an equally experimental anti-nerve agent drug, pyridostig-mine bromide.

The FDA classifies all three of these drugs as investigational new drugs (INDs). Although each had been used on humans before, none were properly tested for efficacy and safety as protective agents against biological/chemical warfare.

The anthrax vaccine is FDA approved for protection from cutaneous (skin) exposure to anthrax spores. Veterinarians and tannery workers have used it for some time, but military weapons disperse anthrax spores via a very fine aerosolized mist that deposits the spores in the lungs through inhalation. A Senate Veterans Affairs Committee report in 1995 concluded that since the vaccine's effectiveness was unknown in the case of inhalation, it should be considered investigational when used as protective agent against bio/chem warfare. As late as August, 1997, a team of Army doctors admitted in the Journal of the American Medical Association that they weren't sure if their vaccine would work.[4]

Botulism is poisoning resulting from a toxin some-

---

[4] "Anthrax and Other Vaccines: Protection or Placebo," *Citizen Soldier* pamphlet.

times found in improperly canned or preserved foods, and can cause muscular paralysis and disturbance of vision and breathing.[5] The safety of the botulism vaccine was not established prior to the Persian Gulf War and remains uncertain. First of all, the existing supply of the vaccine was nearly 20 years old, and there was concern that it would break down into toxic products due to prolonged storage. The FDA conducted tests but did not complete them until January 24, 1991, after the war had started. Secondly, though the test results came back fine, they did not address the problem of adverse reactions previously associated with this vaccine; in 1973 the Center for Disease Control considered terminating its distribution because of adverse reactions.[6]

Pyridostigmine bromide (PB) is a nerve agent pre-treatment, an oral pill to be taken periodically during threat of nerve agent attack.[7] In layman's terms what it does is shut down the peripheral nerve system when it comes in contact with certain nerve agents. It is not an actual treatment for nerve agent poisoning, but a pretreat-ment—a chemical that enhances the effectiveness of two drugs, atropine and 2-PAM, which are proven treatments for nerve agent poisoning.[8]

PB is FDA approved only for treatment of myasthe-nia gravis, a disease of faulty nerve conduction, character-ized by muscular weakness and fatigue.[9] It has never been

---

[5] *Hidden Casualties: The Environmental, Health, and Political Consequences of the Persian Gulf War*, ed. James Warner, Arms Control Research Center, 1994, p. 238.

[6] "Is Military Research Hazardous to Veteran's Health? Lessons Spanning Half A Century," *Committee on Veterans' Affairs* staff report, US Senate, 1994, p. 34.

[7] "Pyridostigmine Used as a Nerve Agent Pretreatment Under Wartime Conditions," Keeler, Hurst, Dunn; JAMA, Aug. 7, 1991, Vol. 266, no. 5, p. 693-5.

[8] "Is Military Research Hazardous to Veteran's Health? Lessons Spanning Half A Century," *Committee on Veterans' Affairs* staff report, US Senate, 1994, p. 11.

[9] *Hidden Casualties: The Environmental, Health, and Political Consequences of the Persian Gulf War*, ed. James Warner, Arms Control Research Center, 1994, p. 238.

properly tested for product safety in healthy individuals. Previous studies involved too few test subjects and virtually excluded women, although 28,000 received dosages during the war. Furthermore, a DOD study conducted just previous to the conflict included extensive safety precautions, including giving medical exams to the men before giving the PB. The researchers indicated that PB should not be given to individuals who suffered from certain conditions. In recognition of known side effects, this study required participants to be in-patients "so that they will be monitored during evening periods of non-testing. A drug will be available at the test site to counteract the possible adverse side effects." The repeated claims that PB is perfectly safe does not mesh with the elaborate safeguards established by researchers. Such safeguards were not taken for the 400,000 service men and women given the drug during the Gulf War.[10]

PB was also never tested for safety in use with other chemical agents that military personnel would be exposed to, namely the insect repellent DEET and the insecticide pemethrin, both used by the Army. In independent studies, researchers at Duke University in Durham, North Carolina and the University of Texas Southwest Medical Center in Dallas, suggest that PB interfered with the body's natural defense against the toxic effects of DEET and Pemethrin, leading to possible nerve damage. In their study researchers exposed chickens to amounts of the chemicals that by themselves were harmless, but when exposed to the chemicals in combination, they began to show signs of nerve damage.[11] The effects of this chemical cocktail could explain a number of the symptoms reported by veterans.

DU is one of the main causes believed to be responsi-

---

[10] "Is Military Research Hazardous to Veteran's Health? Lessons Spanning Half A Century," *Committee on Veterans' Affairs* staff report, US Senate, 1994, p. 29-30.

[11] "Nerve Pill Sapped Soldier's Defences," K. Kleiner, *New Scientist*, April 27, 1996, p. 4.

ble for the sickness known as Gulf War Syndrome, along with the Iraqi Chemical weapons, pollutants from the Kuwaiti oil fires, aerial pesticides sprayed over Saudi Arabia, and non-FDA-approved drugs given to soldiers in case of unconventional weapons attack. Since returning home, thousands of Gulf War soldiers have suffered from muscle spasms, joint and muscle pains, rectal bleeding, respiratory problems, fatigue, headaches, nausea, sleep disorders, weight loss, memory loss, skin rashes, fevers, impotence, miscarriage, and birth defects.[12]

Gulf War Babies

Gulf War veterans know they are sick. The Pentagon denies their sickness, calling them neurotic, and the VA has refused to investigate the cause of their problems. Yet another generation of veterans finds the government whose war they fought has turned its back on them. When a soldier goes to war he or she knows their personal safety is at risk; but what they don't know is that they are risking the lives of their children as well. Perhaps the greatest tragedy of the Gulf War are its tiniest victims. The children of U.S. vets and Iraqis alike are being born deformed, with debilitating and disfiguring conditions that make their little lives unbearable and sometimes impossible.

For vets with afflicted babies, the government runaround can be just as bad as it was for Gulf War Syndrome vets. Military doctors often ignore the signs of birth defects and refuse to speak truthfully with parents. When they do talk they're quick to cite the statistic that at least 3 percent of American babies are born with abnormalities, to which one mother responded: "I'd like to put my child's picture in front of them and say, 'Glance at that once in a while to make sure you're telling me the truth.'" The truth

---

[12] *Hidden Casualties: The Environmental, Health, and Political Consequences of the Persian Gulf War*, ed. James Warner, Arms Control Research Center, 1994, p. 237.

is that the Association of Birth Defect Children (ABDC) have found clustering with certain types of birth defects among children of Gulf War veterans. Clustering is the term epidemiologists use when an ailment strikes one group of people more than others—and the phenomenon can be a key indicator that something more than chance is causing the birth defects.

Gulf War vets and babies also suffer the same cruel indifference from the government in their search for medical assistance. Independent research is complicated by the DOD's reluctance to release information from DU studies. This difficulty is further compounded by the fact that few or inaccurate medical records were kept on the INDs employed during the war. Veterans who know they received experimental vaccines rarely find the inoculations noted in their records, and those who aren't sure are left to guess. Participation in military research is rarely included in military medical records, making it impossible to support a veteran's claim for service-connected disabilities.[13] The government points to the "chaos of war" to excuse this gross oversight.[14]

Goldenhar's syndrome, characterized by a lopsided head and spine, was the first cluster discovered: ten babies with severe cases of a condition that usually strikes one in 26,000, according to ABDC executive director Betty Mekdeci. The ABDC is tracking four more possible clusters. Significantly, not one of the parents from their survey has a family history of these types of birth defects. As Mekdeci puts it, "There have been no relatives with funny ears." Gulf War vets with sick babies face huge medical bills, and the unwillingness of insurance companies to cover preexisting conditions force many to live in poverty

[13] "Is Military Research Hazardous to Veteran's Health? Lessons Spanning Half A Century," *Committee on Veterans' Affairs* staff report, US Senate, 1994, p. 39.
[14] "Military Use of Drugs Not Yet Approved by the FDA for CW/BW Defense," Richard Rettig, RAND report for the Office of the Secretary of Defense, 1999, p. 71.

to qualify for Medicaid. Meanwhile government officials, like Dr. Stephen Joseph, Assistant Secretary of Defense for Health Affairs, make comments that they are entirely unfamiliar with "Goldhavers or Gold Heart—whatever."[15]

Consent

"Drop your shorts, son," said the platoon leader, as the troops lined up in the desert heat, "this baby's your only line of defense against Hussien's arsenal of biological weapons."

"We weren't told it was experimental, we weren't given a choice," says Paul Sullivan, Gulf War veteran. Consent was not an issue.

Under FDA regulations, INDs may be used only with the informed consent of the recipient, but the military was granted a waiver of this rule. After the Iraqi invasion of Kuwait, the FDA bypassed these requirements by issuing a new general regulation. Rule 23(d) declared that consent "is not feasible in a specific military operation involving combat or the immediate threat of combat."[16]

Rule 23(d) raises many ethical questions about human experimentation. Many believe it is a violation of the Fifth Amendment and the Nuremberg code. It was challenged in court by advocacy groups but was upheld when the case went to the Court of Appeals in 1991.[17]

An order issued by General Norman Schwarzkopf that the botulism vaccine was to be given on a voluntary basis, despite the FDA waiver on informed consent, has caused some confusion as to whether the inoculations were voluntary or not. Still, many veterans have complained of forcible administrations of the vaccines. Several testified of such incidents to Citizen Soldier and in a congressional hearing.

---

[15] "The Tiny Victims of Desert Storm," Hudson, Briggs, Miller, *Life.*
[16] *Hidden Casualties: The Environmental, Health, and Political Consequences of the Persian Gulf War,* ed. James Warner, Arms Control Research Center, 1994, p. 239.
[17] ibid.

"They said if I didn't take the vaccination, then I was under UCMJ (Uniform Code of Military Justice) action" or subject to court martial said Philip J. Abbatessa, 101st Airborne Division.

Sgt. Venus Hammack, of Lowell, MA, a veteran with 16 years in the military, told the 1992 House Veterans Affairs Committee that she had been held down and forcibly given the vaccine against her will.

One Army Reserve doctor, Cpt. Yolanda Huet-Vaughn of Kansas City refused to serve in the Gulf, in part because she did not want to vaccinate soldiers without their consent. Sentenced to 30 months, the mother of three was later released after serving 8 months, thanks to pressure from Amnesty International.[18]

A need-to-know basis

Ethical arguments aside, in granting the waiver on consent, the FDA stipulated that the troops should still be properly informed as to the possible effects of the treatments, and required that adequate studies and medical records of doses, inoculations, and any adverse side-effects be maintained. None of this was done. The DOD's entire handling of the INDs was deplorable. The DOD concedes that it did not fulfill its commitment to provide military personnel with information on the hazards posed by experimental drugs used in the Gulf War, information that the FDA considered essential to permit involuntary use.[19]

For example, the FDA normally requires that IND packaging be labeled as experimental. But the military argued that this was misleading since there was no experiment going on (which is questionable and shall be addressed later), and suggested the package be printed with the with the words "for military combat use and eval-

---

[18] ibid.

[19] Comments of Public Citizen Litigation Group to FDA, Sidney Wolfe and Michael Tankersley, Oct. 29, 1997.

uation."[20] The FDA agreed, but when the PB rations were handed out even this ambiguous statement was missing. Later the DOD's own surveys showed that 47% of the military personnel that received PB felt they had received inadequate information.[21]

With an arrogance only the military can achieve, the DOD pointed to Agent Orange as its reason for not informing the troops to the experimental quality of the vaccines and PB. "There was concern among a number of troops we interviewed about possible long term side effects of vaccines and chemotherapeutic prophylactic agents such as pyridostigmine. Rumors were rife and many referred to troop exposure to Agent Orange in Vietnam as a model of their fears." They concluded by citing past instances in which troops had refused to take drugs knowing they were experimental.

"Our judgment is informed by lessons of history."[22]

Agent Orange is hardly the only incident of the military's reckless indifference to the health of its personnel. History proves that the military has long considered its enlistees, and often the unlucky civilian populations near test sites, to be the world's largest pool of human guinea pigs. Some of this research was done with the informed consent of the guinea pigs involved, but these cases are few and far between. The overwhelming majority of history's experiments were carried out on unwitting test subjects who were misinformed, uninformed, or out-and-out lied to. In the case of the mustard gas tests, participants were sworn to secrecy, under threat of imprisonment if they ever discussed these experiments with anyone. Some human experiments were carried out with precise method-

---

[20, 22] *Use of Products Not Approved for General Commercial Marketing for Needed Uses in Military or Civilian Terrorist Exigencies.* Statement included in correspondence from DOD to FDA, Sept. 29, 1997.

[21] From text of Dr. Michael Friedman, Lead Deputy Commissioner—FDA letter to Dr. Edward Martin, Acting Asst. Secretary of Defense for Health Affairs at the Pentagon, July 22, 1997, p. 6.

ology and purpose, like MK-ULTRA. Others, as in the cases of Dugway and the "atomic veterans," were performed with the pure recklessness of a child with a chemistry set but were experiments nonetheless. Are the Gulf War veterans guinea pigs or simply victims? Was the exposure of Desert Storm troops to INDs and DU yet another experiment?

The Answer is Yes

In a rare display of ethical conscience, the army points to the fact it can't very well gas people to check out the efficacy of vaccines or drugs such as PB. What they could do is dose them up, put them in harm's way with a false sense of security, and wait. What they could do is allow them to walk around unprotected in a radioactive dustbin of incinerated DU rounds. They could observe the health effects and make judgment on the practicality of using these drugs and weapons. They could hide behind their show of protecting the troops, pointing to Iraq's noticeable arsenal of bio/chem weapons, all the while conducting their own form of bio/chem warfare on them. It really doesn't matter if they did or didn't keep medical records. Sloppy methodology doesn't equal no experiment. Reckless indifference to the health of a guinea pig doesn't cease to make them human research test subjects. Look to the history. If the military was truly concerned about the safety of the troops, why the carelessness in the application of these drugs—no records, no research, no follow-up...

It appears their only concern was that these drugs would not immediately render soldiers unable to perform their duties. The long-term health effects on personnel and family weren't an issue. Again, look to history. The only object to this "experiment" was to test the efficacy of the INDs in the instance of bio/chem warfare, only Saddam broke the date. "We hanged people at Nuremberg for doing similar things," said Paul Sullivan.

Continued Use of INDs and DU

So the Pentagon, never one to wait by the phone, has moved on to court bigger and better bad guys. Depleted uranium missiles were used in the conflict with Yugoslavia and "accidentally" dumped on Puerto Rico during training maneuvers. All the while, the DOD goes on insisting that somehow this radioactive waste is harmless. The anthrax vaccine is now mandatory for all enlistees, and they have thirty more in the works.

On a brighter note in an otherwise bleak future, the FDA, finding the DOD's handling of the INDs irresponsible, did not grant them the "blanket waiver" to use INDs without informed consent in case or threat of war. Then in October, 1998, Congress passed a bill providing a better health package for Gulf War veterans. Progress can be noted in how the government has been much quicker in responding to Gulf War veterans than it was to notice Vietnam veterans suffering from the effects of Agent Orange. So we can still be poisoned, but at least acknowledgment will be forthcoming. And remember, all you die-hard guinea pigs, when the job market's looking dim, you can always join the Army.

man' slaugh"ter, *n*, The killing of a man or of men by man; homicide; in law, the unlawful killing of another, without malice either expressed or implied. It may be committed voluntarily, as in a sudden passion, or involuntarily, as the result of criminal carelessness, or as an incident in the commission of some wrongful act. Compare HOMICIDE; MURDER. **man' slaugh"** ter- **ous**, *a*.

Cases of *manslaughter* are divided into three classes. (1) Where there was an intent to take life and the killing would be murder but for mitigating circumstances. (2) Where death results from unintentionally doing a unlawful act. (3) Where it results from the negligent doing or omission of an act which, though not itself wrongful, was attended by circumstances which endangered life. Bouvier *Law Dict*. Rawle's revision, vol. ii, p. 308. [Bost. B. Co. 1897.]

Quoted from: *Funk & Wagnalls New Standard Dictionary of the English Language*. New York and London: Funk & Wagnalls Company, 1930

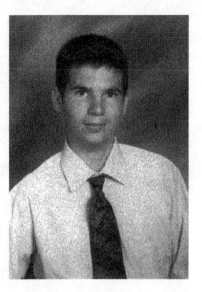

No Charges Filed: The Medical Manslaughter of Jesse Gelsinger
BY ROBERT HELMS

"Clear the air! Clean the sky! Wash the wind! Take the stone from the stone, take the skin from the arm, take the muscle from the bone, and wash them. Wash the stone, wash the bone, wash the brain, wash the soul, wash them wash them!"
—*T. S. Eliot, Murder in the Cathedral, 1935*

Jesse Gelsinger was a bright, optimistic teenager from a working-class family. His father, Paul Gelsinger, makes his living as a handyman. Paul is divorced from Jesse's mother and has re-married, and in the new family's structure Jesse had three siblings. Jesse suffered from a rare enzyme disorder called ornithine transcarbamylase deficiency (OTC). The lack of this enzyme, traceable to a missing gene, interferes with the liver's ability to metabolize ammonia. The fatal form of this ailment usually takes the lives of newborns and children under age 5, but Jesse's case had been managed by thirty-two pills a day and a special low-protein diet. When the young man kept to the course set down by his doctors in Arizona, he enjoyed pretty good health and led a relatively normal life.

In September 1999, Jesse died in a clinical trial aimed at developing a safe treatment for babies who suffer from the more severe form of the disorder. The research was conducted at the University of Pennsylvania in Philadelphia. His case raised many urgent questions about how genetic research is conducted in the United States. Let's switch to a factual timeline gleaned from press reports of the Gelsinger case, after which I will make a few conclusions.

Jesse Gelsinger and the Medical Scientists: A Chronology

1981
June 18: Jesse Gelsinger is born.

1983
Jesse is diagnosed with the non-fatal form of OTC deficiency.

1992
Dr. James M. Wilson founds the private for-profit firm, Genovo, Inc. By 1999 it will annually provide $4.7 million of a $22 million budget to the Institute for Human Gene Therapy at the University of Pennsylvania. Dr. Wilson is a major shareholder of Genovo, as well as the director of the Institute for Human Gene Therapy.

1993
April: Drs. Mark Batshaw and James Wilson begin experiments on OTC deficient mice. They demonstrate the efficacy of the adenovirus as a vector for the OTC gene, but safety studies on mice, rhesus monkeys, and baboons yield mixed results. Three monkeys die from an earlier stronger version of the vector while others suffer severe

hepatitis from the same vector Jesse would receive.

1994

Batshaw and Wilson seek advice from the University's resident bioethics expert, Arthur Caplan, about how to select human subjects for the next phase of the adenovirus research. Caplan advises against using babies dying from OTC deficiency in favor of asymptomatics, adult patients like Jesse. The researchers begin scouting for possible volunteers for clinical trial.

Mid-1995

The Recombinant DNA Advisory Committee of the National Institutes of Health approves the Batshaw-Wilson protocol, with two dissenting experts stating that it is too risky for asymptomatic volunteers. Nineteen OTC-deficient adults eventually enroll in a safety study that gradually increases the dosage in each successive group of three volunteers. This was to determine the maximum safe dosage level for humans. The consent forms they sign do not mention the occurrences of hepatitis and death in the animal experiments. Jesse is in the last group, and will receive the highest dosage planned for the trial.

1998

December: Jesse suffers a severe bout with the disorder after straying from his regimen of medications. He is hospitalized and becomes comatose, but later recovers.

1999

May: Jesse graduates from high school.

June 18: The Gelsinger family flies to Philadelphia for Jesse's screening at the Hospital of the University of Pennsylvania. They take in the tourist sites. It's Jesse's

18th birthday.

June 22: Jesse qualifies for the Batshaw-Wilson study, with a blood ammonia reading of 47 micromoles per deciliter, which is below the maximum of 75 micromoles specified by the protocol. Normal blood ammonia levels are 35 micromoles per deciliter. Jesse is thrilled and returns home to Arizona.

September 9: Jesse flies back to Philadelphia for the adenovirus study. Shortly before leaving, he says to a friend: "What's the worst that can happen to me? I die, and it's for the babies."

September 12: Jesse reports for duty at the university. His blood-ammonia reading is 91 micromoles. Although this reading exceeds the limit set by the protocol, the experiment proceeds.

September 13, 10:30 a.m.: Jesse's hepatic artery is injected with 30 milliliters of the genetically altered adenovirus and he receives medications to reduce the ammonia level in his blood. After two hours, the ammonia reading drops to 60. The surgeon who performs all this work is Dr. Steven E. Raper.

September 14: After the 20th hour of the experiment Jesse develops jaundice (turns yellow) because of a certain clotting disorder that was also previously observed in the dead rhesus monkeys. He sinks into a coma, then into "multiple organ system failure," and is placed on life support.

September 17: Jesse is found to be brain-dead and is removed from life support and pronounced dead. At least nine family members are present.

September 28: The University of Pennsylvania announces that Jesse died as the result of a gene-therapy experiment, and the story is reported worldwide.

October 11: The U.S. Food and Drug Administration forbids any new subjects from entering two ongoing trials similar to the Batshaw-Wilson study, but those already under treatment are allowed to continue.

November 3: *The Washington Post* reports that researchers and drug manufacturers have failed to inform the National Institutes of Health of six deaths that occurred in gene therapy experiments since April 1998.

November 7: Jesse's ashes are scattered by family and friends on Mount Wrightson, near his home in Tucson. They carried his remains in his pill bottles. Dr. Raper is present.

November 9-10: Public hearings are held on Jesse's case at the NIH's headquarters in Bethesda, Maryland. Batshaw, Wilson and Raper begin to admit to discrepancies between the research protocol and their performance, but still defend their conduct. Government officials from the Recombinant DNA Advisory Committee cite the researchers for:

> • Removing language from the consent forms that described the sicknesses and deaths in the earlier animal research;
> • Failing to promptly report severe reactions suffered by two study volunteers at dosages lower than the one Jesse received (they reported this two months later, and proceeded with higher dosages without

consulting the FDA);

- Changing the order of the patients without asking permission (Jesse was second in his set of three, but as the male subject he was supposed to be third);
- Proceeding with the experiment when Jesse's ammonia reading exceeded the maximum allowed by the protocol.

Paul Gelsinger speaks at the hearing, urging all parties to draw positive results from his son's death. Up to this point he has stated that he does not hold the researchers responsible for the tragedy.

2000

January 21: The FDA shuts down all gene therapy experiments at the University of Pennsylvania after finding "numerous serious deficiencies" in the way Jesse's study was run.

January 26: *The New York Times* reports that Paul Gelsinger has hired a lawyer, but that he also wants Batshaw and Wilson to continue with gene therapy research (provided they improve their procedures). The *Times* also reports that the Senate will hold a subcommittee hearing on whether there is sufficient oversight for gene therapy.

January 30: More tardy news comes from Washington: A Harvard-affiliated hospital in Boston suspended a gene-therapy experiment during the summer of 1999 after three of the first six patients died and a seventh fell seriously ill. Reports of 691 serious adverse events in gene therapy experiments have swamped the NIH as a result of the Gelsinger case. Federal rules demand that adverse event reports be filed "immediately" as problems arise, but according to an agency summary requested by Congress, 652 of the 691 had never before been seen by the NIH. This means less than 6% were filed on time. The researchers claim they were unaware of the requirement, even though it is stated clearly on the paperwork that gives approval to every experiment they do.

February 2: Delores Aderman, another volunteer in the Batshaw-Wilson protocol, steps forward. She tells *The Philadelphia Inquirer* that in her case her liver enzymes (levels which serve as gauges for liver cell injury) rose high enough that the researchers reported the toxicity to the Food and Drug Administration, and were then obliged to get permission before proceeding to the next patient. All the doctors told her was that "everything went good."

February 4 & 6: Arthur Caplan and PENN's President write pieces for the *Inquirer* defending their institution without specifically defending the conduct of the Batshaw-Wilson protocol.

February 8: A public panel discussion on genetics and human nature by Wilson and Caplan is held on schedule, but Wilson is replaced at the last minute by a colleague. The facilitator states that Wilson was "unable to make it." Jesse's case is mentioned several times without discussing the breaches of trust involved. Politicians are ridiculed. Caplan showed that he is a highly skilled public speaker, a born comedian, and an apologist for his home team.

Now, let's explore some reasons why this relatively healthy kid was ever strapped to a table, fitted through the groin with arterial catheters, and infused with an experimental gene vector despite blood ammonia readings that should have disqualified him from the procedure. But before we can do that, we must ask who these people at the University of Pennsylvania are:

Arthur L. Caplan is the director of the university's Center for Bioethics, and in recent years has become the most quoted person in his field. He is peculiar because he is a far more visible and more media-friendly spokesperson than any of his peers. Some say he's right in popularizing important discussions, while others say he's just another media whore. In either case, Caplan is a team player, and he does not publicly criticize any researcher who practices under the same roof as he does. In *Guinea Pig Zero* #6, I pointed out his odd silence on the subject of the dermatologist Albert Kligman, who used inmates at Philadelphia's Holmesburg prison as human guinea pigs from the 1950's to the early '70's. In exchange for small cash payments, Kligman tested LSD, dioxin, radioactive isotopes, Agent Orange and poison ivy on Holmesburg inmates. He became very rich (he invented Retin-A) while the inmates underwent excruciating pain and were scarred, went insane and became chronically ill for unknown reasons. When prisoner-experiments came under public scrutiny and Kligman was investigated, he destroyed all his original patient records. There were questions about the dead inmates, but Kligman destroyed the answers with the records. Despite all this, Art Caplan claims no position on whether the surviving inmate guinea pigs should be compensated or otherwise relieved by the university that tortured them. Since the 1998 release of a book documenting Kligman's research, *Acres of Skin*, most everyone else in the city does have a position on this issue. I saw Caplan at a conference on science and religion in the spring of 1999. In passing he remarked that the Holmesburg veterans picketing out on the sidewalk had reached their conclusions by some sort of logical fallacy. No one really understood what he was getting at, but he saved face by giving them a nod. What he did not mention was Kligman's past behavior or the university's refusal to take responsibility for the harm suffered by his living victims.

This bioethics poster-boy was the one who made Jesse's experiment possible by persuading the researchers and government overseers that asymptomatic adult patients should serve as the human subjects, as opposed to infants with fatal cases. He reasoned that parents would be coerced by their babies' sicknesses into putting them at risk. Caplan's letter of February 4, 2000, fiercely defends why adult OTC deficient persons like Jesse should be put at risk even though they were not the intended beneficiaries of the treatment. He also ridiculed a reporter who had taken this up as an issue. The letter's effect was to draw the reader's attention away from the more disturbing facts of the case.

Caplan's name also occurs back in September of 1999, when he argued for an immediate announcement about the nature of Jesse's death. Since then there's been no word on Dr. James M. Wilson's glaring conflict of interests, being both co-author of the experiment's protocol and its prime financial beneficiary, standing to make many millions if the vector proved marketable. It's obvious Caplan knows on which side his ethical bread is buttered.

When a bioethics expert like Arthur Caplan remains silent on such alarming ethical crises, when the players are his colleagues and his own salary and career are controlled by the institution directly vested in the matter, he ceases to serve as an ethics expert and becomes the university's spin doctor. To be sure, he did not directly praise them, but of all people, Caplan is the one whose position should be the clearest and loudest when there is an ethical conflict. Above all, we should keep in mind that he participated in planning the clinical trial that took Gelsinger's life, almost as directly as the researchers themselves.

Next we come to Dr. Mark Batshaw and Dr. Steve Raper. According to a *New York Times* report on Jesse's death, Dr. Batshaw, a pediatrician of great stature, was the scientist hit hardest by the tragedy. The article quoted him as saying that before Jesse he had never made a patient worse by his care. The article also states that he prayed for the dead boy, and thought hard about the Hippocratic Oath; "I did harm," Batshaw said. Also according to the *Times*, Dr. Steve Raper has "thrown himself into his work" and committed himself to finding the treatment the experiment was intended to find so this loss of life will not be in vain. As he pronounced Gelsinger dead, Dr. Raper said, "Goodbye, Jesse. We'll figure this out." Later, he pondered whether the vector had reacted badly with Jesse's medications or if the reactions in the rhesus monkeys had meant more than he realized.

As it happens I'm wondering the same things, and experts are publicly discussing the matter. For example, geneticist Robert Malone of the University of Maryland told the *Inquirer* that "There was adequate literature to show the adenovirus was a problem—even from [animal studies in] Wilson's own lab. The writing was on the wall for five years."

Dr. Raper is the surgeon who physically performed the experiment on Jesse Gelsinger, and who agreed to proceed with the infusion even though Jesse's ammonia levels exceeded the allowed maximum at the beginning of the experiment. Drs. Batshaw and Raper interpreted "day of enrollment" as different from "day of the treatment," and they did not let the lines of safety interfere with the ambitious experiment. Let's remember that Batshaw co-wrote the protocol; he believed 75 micromoles was the safe limit, and he wrote that into the protocol. Why would he bend his own rule less than three months later when Jesse

NO CHARGES FILED: THE MEDICAL MANSLAUGHTER OF JESSE GELSINGER arrived with 91 micromoles? Those kinds of levels weren't just over the stated limit, they were nearly double the reading of 47 that Jesse showed when he first enrolled. Why did Dr. Raper agree to go ahead with the experiment? Did he explain his decision to Jesse?

The answer, I believe, lies with Dr. James M. Wilson. This man is not just a physician, he's also a financial investor. With Jesse strapped in and catheterized in a hospital room in West Philadelphia, Wilson was almost done with an experiment that would make him very rich and world-famous. After his great experiment proved fatal for Jesse, he aired his feelings to *New York Times* journalist Sheryl Gay Stolberg about whether he should have done anything differently: "At this point, I say no, but I'm continuing to re-evaluate constantly." The journalist continues, describing Wilson as "besieged by worry, about the morale of his staff, about whether his financial sponsors would pull out, about whether patients would continue to volunteer, about whether he would lose his bravado—the death knell for a scientist on the cutting edge.

"'My concern,' Wilson confessed, over dinner one night in Philadelphia, 'is, I'm going to get timid, that I'll get risk averse.'"

Let's remember that *The New York Times* is not a confrontational paper, nor is it the least bit radical. When its reporter asked Wilson how he felt, she was not trying to set him up, nor would her editors have been likely to print any embarrassing quotes had she submitted any. We live in an age when major publications are terribly afraid of being sued and almost never take chances with muckraking articles on powerful institutions like the University of Pennsylvania.

Dr. James Wilson was not embarrassed to say that he has a clear business interest in the experiment that cost Gelsinger his life. He also did not admit remorse for the risks he subjected his patient to, but for the chance his business life will be harmed by Jesse's death. With the smell of a dead guinea pig following him around, he won't be half the scientific cowboy we've all grown to love.

I am led to the conclusion that Drs. Wilson, Batshaw and Raper put Jesse Gelsinger at more risk than they knew to be safe because they stood to make significant financial and career gains from the reckless adventure. However, it's clear enough that only Wilson is oblivious to the problem.

Finally, who am I to say that Jesse was not mature enough to decide if this experiment was a safe risk? Who am I to contradict Jesse's father, who until recently has refused to turn against the researchers at all, who still holds them essentially blameless, and who wishes to portray Jesse's sacrifice in the most positive light? There are a few points I can consider:

I was reminded of my own youth when I read descriptions of Jesse's heroic attitude as he went to war against his disease. Before Jesse was born, I joined the Navy and walked into boot camp to have my head shaved on my 18th birthday, Jesse's age when he first arrived in Philadelphia. Had I been a few years older, I wouldn't have done that. As I matured, I became less easy to persuade. I'm lucky I didn't have to die, but Jesse never should have.

I also have a special concern that Paul Gelsinger does not have—I personally volunteer my own body for medical experiments. Every time I do this, I sign a consent form just like Jesse did. Every time I sign, I base my consent on the information on the form and usually nothing else. Drs. Batshaw and Wilson deliberately altered the consent form to soften the facts. They removed the reports of hepatitis and death in rhesus monkeys so Jesse and Paul Gelsinger wouldn't be alarmed. If they get away with this deceit, I'll have to swallow very hard the next time I put my pen to a consent form. I'll have to look carefully into the eyes of the doctor as he or she hands me the little plastic cup with the capsule lying in it; are his thoughts like my thoughts? Where is his money? Do I see ambition in that steady stare? Does a human heart beat under that lab coat, or is this a lizard, clawing at a financial pipeline with one hand and clinging to the flesh of my arm with the other?

There is another way this story touches home for me: Jesse was not only a fellow human guinea pig, he was the son of a fellow handyman. A handyman is a guy who looks for jobs and then has them come to him on the merits of his past performances. Either he is reliable and trustworthy or he starves. I know the eye contact between handyman and customer when they say "Here are the keys to my house." Paul Gelsinger is a handyman who was convinced by three Ivy League scientists that his boy was safe in their hands. He now sees that he was wrong to trust them and that they were operating from a position of enormous advantage.

The media's treatment of Jesse's doctors has been quite mild, and until shortly before this piece the government has been cautious. Once again the Congress is planning a subcommittee hearing, but I am underwhelmed by the shallow courage of our elected leaders. First there was Senator Glenn's bill that went nowhere. Representative Shays' initiative also went nowhere. Here comes another round with Jesse's name all over it, and what's coming out of the National Institutes of Health and the Office for Protection from Research Risks sounds good. However, until I'm proven wrong, I'll hold that this government lacks the power and the political will to demand researchers to disclose everything to their subjects and to respect the subject's safety as much as their own. There are simply too many dollars and too many Arthur Caplans on the Industry Team. The NIH is currently showing us they care in a bureaucratic way, but they have yet to force doctors to even be aware of what the rules are. There will never be laws that researchers will fear like any other guys peddling drugs to neighbor's kids. Researchers lie to subjects and grow rich, but they fear no jail and no handcuffs. Bad press and loss of face is the worst it ever gets.

I expect to hear a little discussion of tightened regulations and better federal oversight for genetic research, but not much else. Should Paul Gelsinger bring a lawsuit, and I sure hope he does, money will change hands and all parties will fall silent forever. Also, I hope that Mr. Gelsinger will not allow himself to be seduced again, this time with statues, memorial lecture series, scholarships named for his son, and so on. But Paul's statements in the *Times* worries me that he may do just that: "they should not be put out of business ... I don't want to see anybody lose their job ... "

Jesse Gelsinger died trying to do the world some good, and three researchers walked him to his death trying to be first to find another profitable scientific breakthrough. Such is life and death for an honest young man in the medical marketplace.

Goodbye, Jesse. We'll keep an eye on those bastards.

Jesse's Intent
BY PAUL GELSINGER

Born on June 18, 1981, Jesse Gelsinger was a real character in a lot of ways. We hadn't picked a name before he was born, but the name Jesse came to us three days later. When considering a middle name, we pondered James, but decided that just Jesse was enough for this kid. His infancy was pretty normal. With a brother 13 months his senior he was not overly spoiled. He crawled and walked at the appropriate ages. When he started talking, it quickly became obvious that this was one kid that would speak his mind and crack everybody up. He nursed until he was nearly two years old. It wasn't until he was about 2 years and 8 months old that his metabolic disorder reared its ugly head. Jesse had always been a very picky eater. Since weaning, he increasingly refused to eat meat and dairy products, focusing instead on potatoes and cereals. After the birth of his sister in late January, 1984, and following a mild cold earlier that March, Jesse's behavior turned briefly erratic and his speech became belligerent. Since his mother had previously experienced schizophrenic behavior, I was very concerned that Jesse was exhibiting signs of psychosis. My wife Pattie and I took him to see our family doctor. He put Jesse on a high protein diet, thinking his poor diet and lethargy may have lead to anemia. That was actually the worst thing for Jesse's condition; forcing him to eat peanut butter sandwiches, bacon and to drink milk over the next two days overwhelmed Jesse's system.

On a Saturday in mid-March, 1984, Jesse awoke, parked himself in front of the television to watch cartoons, and promptly fell back asleep. We became alarmed when we were unable to rouse him. His mother called the doctor and insisted that we take Jesse to the Children's Hospital of Philadelphia, just across the Delaware River from our home near Woodbury, New Jersey. Upon arrival at CHOP, Jesse was admitted through the emergency room. He was in what they called a first stage coma. He responded to stimuli but would not awaken. After several tests indicated high blood ammonia, the doctor told us that Jesse most probably had Reye's syndrome, which upset us very much. Several hours and more tests later they told us it actually wasn't Reye's, and that more tests were needed. Within a week we had the diagnosis of ornithine transcarbamylase deficiency syndrome (OTC), a very rare metabolic disorder caused by a missing gene that creates a needed enzyme. Jesse's form of the disorder was considered mild and could be controlled by medication and diet.

Jesse came home after eleven days in the hospital, and we watched everything he ate like hawks and made certain he took his medications. From there on Jesse progressed fairly normally, although he was small for his age. It wasn't until he was 10 that he would again need to be hospitalized for his disorder. Following a weekend of too much protein, Jesse's system couldn't rid itself of the ammonia buildup fast enough, and he again slipped into a coma. His specialist had never had to treat hyperammonemia before and scrambled to get him well again. Within five days Jesse was well enough to go home, having suffered no apparent neurological damage.

As Jesse entered his teenage years he resisted taking his medications. He felt that he could control his disorder and only took his meds when he didn't feel well. His mother and I had divorced in 1989, two years after our move to Tucson, Arizona. I had obtained custody of my four children in 1990, so Jesse was under my care. At age 16 Jesse was taking nearly fifty pills a day to control his illness. I had remarried in 1992, and my new wife Mickie and I kept a careful watch on him, but as he grew older we expected him to take more responsibility for his own care. With six children between us we had much to consider. Jesse was being seen at a state-funded metabolic clinic in Tucson twice a year to monitor his development, and while not always compliant, he was progressing into adulthood.

In September, 1998, Jesse's specialist told us of a clinical trial being done at the University of Pennsylvania in Philadelphia. They were working on what he described as "gene therapy" for Jesse's disorder. We were instantly interested, but Jesse needed to be an adult to participate, so he was told he had to wait until he was 18. That same fall Jesse was stressing his metabolism like never before, having recently acquired a part time job and an off-road motorcycle, and as a senior in high school he had a very busy schedule. Jesse was having symptoms of his disorder at the time but was trying to hide them—he didn't want restrictions placed on him due to his disorder. I knew he was inconsistent in taking his medications because I rarely had to re-order them. I spoke with him every other week about his need to take better care of himself, but it took his nearly dying to wake him up.

On December 22, 1998, I arrived home in mid-afternoon to find Jesse curled up on the couch. A close friend was with him and Jesse was very frightened. He was vomiting uncontrollably and could not hold down his medications. After about five minutes I determined I couldn't manage his recovery and convinced his pediatrician and specialist that Jesse needed to be hospitalized and placed on intravenous fluids. With his ammonia levels at six times the normal, Jesse was in trouble. No significant changes occurred in his condition by December 24, so the hospital let him go home for Christmas. Jesse was listless all day and crashed Christmas night. He was admitted to intensive care where they discovered hypoglycemia, or seriously low blood sugar. His specialist felt certain that it was due to one of his medications, l-arginine, and discontinued it. He also decided that Jesse's primary medication, sodium benzoate, was not effective enough and ordered that a newer, better medication be provided.

Jesse recovered well enough to be placed in a regular room at the hospital, but his ammonia levels refused to drop. I stayed in the hospital at Jesse's side day and night. Two days after Christmas, on a Sunday afternoon, Jesse and I had a conversation about how he was doing. It seemed that he was stuck up a tree, I said to him, not knowing whether he was going to climb down or fall out. I went home to be with the rest of my family and sleep in my own bed for one night. Jesse called me at about 11:00 p.m. and said, "Dad, I fell out of the tree." He was vomiting uncontrollably again. I rushed back to the hospital and spent a heartrending two days trying to help my son through his crisis. On Monday I learned that the insurance company was balking at new medication payments, so the meds had not been shipped. I told the pharmacist to purchase the new medications with my credit card ($3300 for one month's supply) and that I would deal with the insurance company later. At that point the insurance company relented and authorized the medications that Tuesday, December 29, but by Tuesday afternoon Jesse was so listless I was afraid he wouldn't get well.

At 5:00 p.m. Jesse's vomiting returned and he became incoherent. I went into the hall for help and found his pediatrician examining his chart. While the pediatrician called in the intensive care doctor I called my wife and told her to come immediately. Jesse's aunt and grandmother arrived for a visit only to find Jesse in a crisis. Mickie arrived and together we held Jesse while they prepared a bed for him in intensive care. The ICU doctor, seeing Jesse's deteriorating condition and believing him mentally impaired, inquired if life support would be appropriate. It was then that I realized these people did not know Jesse at all, and I explained that his lack of mental faculties was not his normal state. Jesse developed tremors and began to vomit, then he just stopped. I whispered to Mickie, "He's still breathing, isn't he?" I asked Jesse's pediatrician to check him. After placing his stethoscope on Jesse's chest for a few moments he looked to the nurse and told her to call a code blue. We were whisked from the room while they intubated and manually ventilated Jesse and then took him to intensive care. We were distraught and believed Jesse was near death. After 15 minutes they indicated that they were getting him under control and that his heart never stopped.

For two days Jesse lingered in an induced coma while a ventilator controlled his breathing. He weighed only 97 pounds, down from his healthy weight of 120. His old medication only partially lowered his ammonia level. On Thursday morning Jesse's new medications had arrived, and the doctors gave them to him along with a special nutritional formula through a gastrointestinal feed. Within 24 hours Jesse's ammonia levels started falling. We waited at his side as he began to regain consciousness, and his first conscious act was to motion for us to change the television station—Jesse was back. Within a day he was out of intensive care with normal ammonia levels, something he had never known his entire life. He was now ordering and eating food like a teenager—again, something he had never before experienced. We were ecstatic. When his specialist came I shook his hand and told him that he had a medical miracle on his hands. A week after nearly dying Jesse was back in school full-time with a new-found zeal for life.

By early February, 1999, Jesse had recovered enough strength to consider returning to work, but then came down with a serious case of influenza. Illness often triggered Jesse's metabolic disorder, so I stayed home to keep an eye on his condition. Jesse recovered within a week and was back in school. I had him tested twice while he was ill and his ammonia levels rose only slightly; the new meds were working wonderfully. He was also kind enough to pass the bug on to me; it was the sickest I'd been in twenty years, with a fever for six days and fatigue for four weeks.

Near the end of that February Jesse returned to his part-time job as a courtesy clerk at a supermarket. On Saturday the 27th he called me at 11:00 p.m. for a ride home. I picked him up in my work van and on the way home we had a fateful conversation. I had been asking Jesse to find out if his job would offer him medical insurance once he graduated from school that May. Being a typical teenager he had done nothing to inquire, and I told him in no uncertain terms that he needed medical insurance if he didn't intend to continue his education. At the time we believed Jesse would not be covered under our insurance once he left school. He rarely raged at his illness, but this time he flung a half-full bottle of soda against my windshield while cursing his disorder. I angrily gave him a backhand punch to the shoulder and chastised him. We were only two blocks from home when Jesse flung open the door and told me he was jumping out. "Whoa, wait until I stop," I said, but before I could come to a stop he gave me a look like he was jumping and out the door he went. All I could envision was Jesse falling under the van and me running him over. Sure enough, even though I had nearly stopped, he fell, and then I could hear him screaming that I was on his arm. Now, my van is a work van loaded with tools and weighs six thousand pounds. 'Oh God, No!' I thought as I threw the van in park and raced around the back of the van to find Jesse's right arm and elbow pinned under my right rear tire. I made certain that his body was clear and rolled the van forward off his arm. The kid was crying in agony. As I cradled him in my arms, I cried, "You idiot, what were you thinking," and "Jesse, I'm sorry." I knew he would need an ambulance. His arm was a red mess from wrist to upper arm with his elbow area gouged out. The tire print was evident on the underside of his arm. A woman who had witnessed what happened while driving asked if she could help, and I asked her to please call 911. A neighbor, hearing the commotion, came out and offered his help. Another passerby offered me his cell phone and I called my wife. Within minutes the paramedics arrived, strapped Jesse to a gurney and whisked him off to the hospital. The police informed me that I had done no wrong, that I could not control his actions, but it was all I could do to drive the one block left home. I had been there to help Jesse through his near death experience in December and through a serious flu only to nearly end his life in an accident.

I was shaking and emotional as my wife Mickie drove me to the hospital. Jesse was okay—he hadn't even broken his arm! He did suffer extensive road rash and a serious wound to his elbow, but he recovered full use of his arm following two days in the hospital and a month of physical therapy. I was an emotional wreck the week following the accident; this kid was something else. His sister told him that if he caused me to have a heart attack she was going to kill him. A month later I got word from our insurance company regarding Jesse's status if he did not continue his education. He was covered until age 25 as long as he remained our dependent. I joked with him that I had run him over for nothing. He was proud of his war wound with dad. God, what a relief it was to see this kid bounce back again.

In early April 1999, Jesse had another appointment at the metabolic clinic. While there, the subject of gene therapy and the clinical trial at the University of Pennsylvania came up again. Jesse and I were both still very intrigued. I informed the doctor that we were already planning a trip to New Jersey in late June, that Jesse would be 18 at that time, and to let Penn know we were interested. I received a letter from Penn in late April firming things up, and by late May our visit was set. We would fly in on June 18 and he would be tested on the 22. Jesse was none too happy about flying in on the 18; that was his birthday and he wanted to party with his friends, but a few days later he told me it was okay. That was good since I'd already bought all six of us tickets a month earlier.

So on Friday, June 18, 1999, Jesse, his three siblings PJ (age 19), Mary (15), and Anne (14), Mickie and I boarded a plane to take us down a path we never imagined. We had a party for Jesse that night at my brother's house. We had a reunion with ten of my fifteen siblings and their extended families that Sunday. It was great to see everyone. The kids got to meet cousins they hadn't seen in 12 years. Jesse's cousins nicknamed him Captain Kirk for the way he struck the volleyball with a two-handed chop. This was turning into a great vacation.

We hung out on Monday and on Tuesday, June 22, we all headed over to Philly to meet with the clinical trial people. We arrived late because of a wrong turn on the expressway only to find that they weren't ready for us. The nurse in charge rounded up Dr. Raper, one of the study's heads, and after a 45-minute wait we were ushered into a hospital room to discuss the procedures and go over consent forms. Dr. Raper described the technique to be used: Jesse would be sedated and two catheters would be placed into his liver; one catheter would inject the viral vector in the hepatic artery at the inlet to the liver, and the other would monitor the blood exiting the liver to assure the organ was absorbing the entire vector. He explained the attendant dangers, and told us Jesse would need to remain immobile for about eight hours after the infusion to minimize the risk of a clot breaking free from the infusion site. Dr. Raper also explained that Jesse would get flu-like symptoms for a few days, and that there was a remote possibility of hepatitis. When I asked about this he explained that hepatitis was just an inflammation of the liver and that the liver was a remarkable organ, the only one in the body with the ability to regenerate itself. While reading the consent form I noticed the possibility of a liver transplant being required if the hepatitis progressed. Hepatitis seemed such a remote possibility and the need for a transplant so rare that no alarms went off in my head. Dr. Raper proceeded to the next phase and what appeared to be the most dangerous aspect of the test—a needle biopsy was to be performed on Jesse's liver one week after the infusion. There would be no benefit to Jesse, Dr. Raper explained; even if the genes worked, the effect would be transient because the body's immune system would attack and kill the virus over a 4-6 week period. Numbers explaining the risks of uncontrolled side effects were also included—there was a one in ten thousand chance that Jesse could die of the biopsy. I said to Jesse that he needed to read and understand what he was getting into, that this was serious stuff. The risks seemed very remote but very real. Still, to my mind one in ten thousand weren't bad odds.

After our 45-minute conversation with Dr. Raper, Jesse consented to undergo the 5-hour N15 ammonia study to determine his level of enzyme efficiency. Many vials of blood were taken before Jesse drank a small vial of

N15 ammonia. This special isotope of ammonia would then show up in Jesse's blood and urine, and the rate at which it was processed out of the body would determine Jesse's efficiency. Going into this study we were aware that Jesse's efficiency was only 6% of a normal person. After waiting with Jesse for two hours we all decided to head out to Pat's Steaks for lunch and to tour South Street for a few hours. On our return to the hospital, Jesse was done and ready to go. It was now mid-afternoon, and we decided to see the Betsy Ross house and Independence Mall. After checking out the Liberty Bell the kids wanted to see the Rocky statue, so we headed over to the Art Museum. Four of us, Jesse, PJ, Mary and me, raced up the steps Rocky-style (we had watched the movie the night before); we only found Rocky's footsteps because the statue had been moved to the Spectrum, so we headed over to Pattison Avenue. A Phillies' game was about to start, so I stayed in our rented Durango while Mickie took pictures of the kids. It was a fun time for everyone, especially Jesse. He was starting to feel good about what he was doing. This was his thing, and he had a chance to help others by it. The following day we toured New York City. Everybody got to pick a place to visit. Jesse chose FAO Schwartz toy store, where he bought four Pro Wrestling action figures. We all had a great day, finishing with the Empire State Building and the Staten Island Ferry.

Four weeks later, back in Tucson, we received a letter addressed to Mr. Paul Gelsinger and Jesse. It was from Dr. Mark Batshaw confirming Jesse's 6% efficiency of OTC and stating that they would like to have Jesse in their study. I presented the letter to Jesse and asked him if he still wanted to do this. He hesitated for a moment, then said yes. Dr. Batshaw called about a week later to follow up his letter and briefly spoke to Jesse, who told the doctor that he would need to call back and explain everything to me; Jesse was deferring to me for understanding this whole thing, and Dr. Batshaw was well aware of that. When I spoke to the doctor we discussed a number of things. He faxed us the graph showing Jesse's N15 results because they forgot to include the graph in the letter. I asked if Jesse was the least efficient patient in the study, and Dr. Batshaw said he was. The doctor then steered the conversation to the results they had experienced to date, explaining they had shown the treatment had temporarily worked in mice, even preventing death in mice exposed to lethal injections of ammonia. He then explained that the most recent patient had shown a 50% increase in her ability to excrete ammonia following gene therapy. "Wow Mark! This really works," I said. "So, with Jesse at 6% efficiency you may be able to show exactly how well this works." His response was that was their hope, and that it would be for these kids. He explained there were another twenty-five liver disorders that could be treated with same technique, and overall these disorders affect one in about every 500 people. I did some quick math and figured that's 500,000 people in the U.S.A. alone and 12,000,000 worldwide. I dropped my guard. Dr. Batshaw and I never discussed the dangerous side of this work. When I told Jesse what Mark Batshaw had to say he knew the right thing to do; he signed on to help everybody and, hopefully, himself. The plan was for him to be the last patient tested, and he was tentatively scheduled for mid-October.

So by late July, 1999, Jesse had a new focus for his life, but he also had other priorities. I had just bought him a used street motorcycle as a graduation present and he was getting his driver's license in August. It was so great to see him grinning ear to ear as he drove drive off on his bike for the first time. He had also just gotten a tattoo on the back of his right calf. Of course, he didn't discuss this with me first and he used money he owed me to get it done. We saw little of Jesse over the next two weeks. If he wasn't working he was out riding with his buddy Gar or spending the night at a friend's house. He was still living at home and paying $35 a week for rent and $15 a week for the bike insurance we fronted for him. This kid was really living and we were proud of him.

In mid-August we heard from Penn that they were having trouble scheduling their next patient and were wondering if Jesse would be available in September. I checked with Jesse, and he ok'd it and arranged an unpaid leave of absence. The finalized date of admission would be September 9, 1999. I wanted to go with Jesse, but being self-employed and not seeing any great danger, I scheduled to fly in for what I thought would be the most dangerous aspect of the testing, the liver biopsy. I would fly in on the 18 and return with Jesse on the 21.

As the date approached we all became more focused on Jesse's trip. Mickie bought him some new clothes, Jesse assembled his pro wrestling, Sylvester Stallone, and Adam Sandler videos, and I worked like a dog to get as much done as possible before my own departure. So with a bag of videos and a bag of clothing, Jesse and I headed off to the airport early that Thursday, September 9. He was both apprehensive and excited. He had to change planes in Phoenix and hail a cab for the hospital once he arrived in Philly. Jesse had never been away from Tucson on his own before this trip. Words cannot express how proud I was of this kid. Just 18, he was going off to help the world. I walked him to his gate, gave him a big hug, looked him in the eye and told him he was my hero. As I drove off to work I thought of him and what he was doing and started considering how to get him some recognition. Little did I know what an effect this kid was going to have.

Jesse called us that night using his phone card. He was well, but had a little mix-up with the cabbie about which hospital to go to, but said the cabbie was cool about it. Jesse was to have more N15 testing the following day and again on Sunday before the actual gene infusion on Monday, September 13. Saturday was an off day so he could leave the hospital. Two of my brothers had arranged to visit with him and that put me at ease. Jesse had a blast with his uncle and cousins on Saturday and a good visit with his other uncle and aunt that Sunday. Mickie and I spoke with Jesse every day and his spirits were good, but he was apprehensive on Sunday evening. Dr. Raper had put him on intravenous medications because his ammonia was elevated. I reasoned with him that these guys knew what they were doing, that they knew more about OTC than anybody on the planet, but it was late so I didn't talk with the doctors.

I received a call from Dr. Raper that Monday just after they infused Jesse. He explained that everything went well and that Jesse would return to his room in a few hours. We discussed the infusion and how the vector did its job. Dr. Raper didn't like the word 'invade' when I explained what I thought the virus did to the liver cells. He explained that if they could affect only about one percent of Jesse's cells they would get the results they desired. Mickie and I spoke with Jesse later that evening. He had the expected fever and was not feeling well. I told him to hang in there and that I loved him. "I love you too, dad," he responded. Mickie got the same kind of goodbye. We didn't know it would be our last.

I awoke very early Tuesday morning and went to work. I received a mid-morning call from Steve Raper asking if Jesse had a history of jaundice. I told him not since he was first born. He explained that Jesse was jaundiced and a bit disoriented. "That's a liver function, isn't it?" I asked. He replied it was and that they would keep me posted. I was alarmed and worried. My ex-wife Pattie happened to call about twenty minutes later; I told her what was going on and she reminded me that Jesse had jaundice for three weeks at birth. I called Penn back with that information and got somebody who was apparently typing every word I said. That seemed very unusual to me. I didn't hear from the doctors again until mid-afternoon. Dr. Batshaw called and said Jesse's condition was getting worse, that his blood ammonia was rising and that he was in trouble. When I asked if I should get on a plane he said to wait, that they were running another test. He called back an hour and a half later and said Jesse's ammonia had doubled to 250 micromoles per deciliter. I told him I was on a plane and would be there in the morning.

It's a very helpless feeling knowing your kid is in serious trouble and you're a continent away. My plane was delayed out of Tucson but got into Philly at 8:00 a.m. Arriving at the hospital at 8:30 I immediately went to find Jesse. As I entered the surgical intensive care I noted a lot of activity in the first room I passed. I waited at the nurse's station for perhaps a minute before announcing who I was. Immediately, Drs. Batshaw and Raper approached me and asked to talk in a private conference room. They explained that Jesse was on a ventilator and in a coma, that his ammonia had peaked at 393 micromoles per deciliter (that's at least ten times a normal reading), and that they were just completing dialysis and had his levels down under 70. They explained that he was having a blood-clotting problem and that because he was breathing above the ventilator and hyperventilating his blood ph was too high. They wanted to induce a deeper coma to allow the ventilator to breath for him. I gave my ok and went in to see my son.

After dressing in scrubs, gloves and a mask because of the isolation requirement, I tried to see if I could rouse my boy. Not a twitch, nothing. I was very worried, especially when the neurologist expressed her concern at the way that his eyes were downcast; not a good sign, she said. When the intensivist told me that the clotting problem was going to be a real battle, I grew even more concerned. I called and talked to my wife, crying and afraid for Jesse. It was at least as bad as the previous December, only this time they had been in his liver. I would keep her posted.

They got Jesse's breathing under control and his blood ph back to normal. The clotting disorder was described as improving and Dr. Batshaw returned to Washington DC by mid-afternoon. I started to relax, believing Jesse's condition was improving. My brother and his wife arrived at the hospital around 5:30 p.m. and we went out for dinner. When I returned I found Jesse in a different intensive care ward. As I sat watching his monitors I noted his oxygen content dropping. The nurse saw me noticing and asked me to wait outside, explaining that the doctors were returning to examine Jesse. At 10:30 p.m. Dr. Raper explained that Jesse's lungs were failing and they were unable to oxygenate his blood even on 100% oxygen. "Whoa, don't you have some sort of artificial lung?" I asked. He thought about it for a moment and said yes, but he would need to call in the specialist to see if Jesse was a candidate. I told him to get on it. I called my wife and told her to get on a plane immediately. At 1:00 a.m. Dr. Raper and the specialist Dr. Shapiro indicated that Jesse had about a 10% chance of survival on his own and 50% with an artificial lung called an ECMO unit. Hooking up the unit would involve inserting a large catheter into the jugular to get a large enough blood supply. I said, "50% is better than 10, let's do it." It seemed like forever for them to even get the ECMO unit ready. Jesse's oxygen levels were crashing. At 3:00 a.m., as they were about to hook Jesse up, Dr. Shapiro rushed into the waiting room to tell me that Jesse was in crisis and rushed back to work on him. The next few hours were really tough. I didn't know anything. Anguish, despair, every emotion imaginable went through me. At 5:00 a.m. Dr. Shapiro came back and said they had the ECMO working, but there was a major leak and Dr. Raper had his finger on it. I quipped that I was a bit of a plumber, if that's what they needed. Shapiro returned to work on Jesse and I began to worry for my wife; Hurricane Floyd hit North Carolina at 3:00 a.m. and was heading toward Philly. I entered the intensive care area at 7:00 a.m. after noting four people still working on Jesse and another half-dozen observing. I approached the nurses station and asked if they could check with the airport to see if my wife would get in ok. They agreed to check and asked if I would like a chaplain. I'm a pretty tough guy, but it was time for spiritual help. At first they sent a young woman who I think was Jewish. I guess she felt a bit out of place since I'm a Christian, and another chaplain, a Christian man a few years younger than me was called in to help. At this point I was trying to contact my family, my mother, for emotional support. A hospital staffer was very helpful in that respect.

By mid-morning six of my siblings and their spouses had arrived. Mickie's plane got in just before they closed the airport and she took a taxi to the hospital. We weren't able to see Jesse until after noon. Dr. Batshaw was stuck on a train that was disabled by the hurricane. Drs. Raper and Shapiro described Jesse's condition as very grave; whatever reaction his body was having would have to subside before he could recover. His lungs were severely damaged and if he survived it would be a very lengthy recovery. They had needed more than ten units of blood in hooking him up. When we finally got to see Jesse he was bloated beyond recognition. The only way to be sure it was Jesse was the battle scar with his dad on his elbow and the tattoo on his right calf. My siblings were shaken to the core. Mickie touched him ever so gently and lovingly. Our hearts nearly broke.

With the hurricane closing in and threatening to close the bridges home, my siblings left by late afternoon. My sister and her husband stayed to take us to dinner and drive us, exhausted, to our hotel. After sleeping for an hour, I arose and felt compelled to return to Jesse. I left Mickie a note and walked the half-mile back to the hospital in a light rain. Hurricane Floyd had skirted Philly and was heading out to sea. Jesse's condition was no better. I noted blood in his urine. 'How can anybody survive this?!' I thought. I said a quiet goodbye to Jesse and returned to the hotel at about 11:30 p.m. I found Mickie preparing to join me. I described his condition as no different and returned to bed. Mickie went out walking for a couple hours.

We arrived at Jesse's room at 8:00 a.m. A new nurse indicated that the doctors wished to speak to us in an hour or so about whether they should continue with their efforts. We went to have breakfast at the hospital cafeteria. Mickie wanted to believe he would get well, but I told her we should be prepared for a funeral. Drs. Batshaw and Raper were there when we returned. They told us that Jesse had suffered irreparable brain damage and that his vital organs were all shutting down. They wanted to shut off life support. They left us alone for a few minutes and we collapsed into each other. On their return I told them I wanted to bring my family in for a brief service prior to ending Jesse's life. Then I told them that they would be doing a complete autopsy to determine why Jesse had died, that this should not have happened. Waves of anger toward the doctors swept over me as I waited for my siblings, but I said to myself, "No, they couldn't have seen this." I went so far as to tell Dr. Batshaw that I didn't blame them and would never file a lawsuit. Little did I know what they really knew.

Seven of my siblings, their spouses and one of my nieces were present for Jesse's brief ceremony, which was at this point more for us. I had all the monitors shut off in his room. Leaning over Jesse, I turned and declared to everyone present that Jesse was a hero. I signaled the doctors after the chaplain's final prayer. Dr. Shapiro clamped off Jesse's blood flow to the ECMO machine and shut off the ventilator. After the longest minute of my life, Dr. Raper stepped in and I removed my hand from Jesse's chest. After listening with a stethoscope for a moment he said, "Goodbye, Jesse, we'll figure this out." Not a dry eye all around. This kid died about as pure as it gets. I was humbled beyond words. My kid had just shown me what it was really all about. I still feel that way.

I supported these doctors for months, believing that their intent was nearly as pure as Jesse's was. Even after the media started exposing flaws in their work I supported them. I had discovered that federal supervision was woefully inadequate, that many researchers were not reporting adverse reactions, and that the FDA was being influenced to inaction by industry. I decided to attend the Recombinant DNA Advisory Committee meeting in December where all the experts were to discuss my son's death. It wasn't until that three-day meeting that I discovered how little efficacy there could be in humans. I had believed this therapy was working based on my conversations with Mark Batshaw, and this is why I defended Penn for so long. These men could not go in front of their peers at the Recombinant DNA Advisory Committee meeting in Bethesda and say the study was working. After Penn and the FDA made their presentations on December 9, I asked for a lunch meeting with the FDA, NIH and the Penn doctors. After touching on many issues I let them all know that I had not yet spoken to a lawyer, but would be in the near future. Too many mistakes had been made and unfortunately, because of our litigious society, it was the only way to correct these problems.

There is so much more to Jesse's story. I can't help but believe that they will kill this with time and money, as they always seem able to do. Who are "they?". They are the heartless and soulless industry and their lobbying efforts; they are the politicians more interested in placating industry than in protecting the people; they are doctors so blinded in their quest for recognition that they no longer see the dangers. Let them apply Jesse's intent to their efforts, and then they'll get it right.

LITERATURE

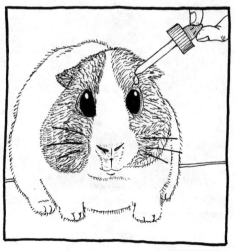

ILLUSTRATION BY DUG

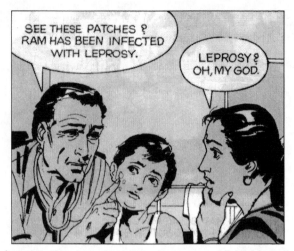

An educational comic strip on Leprosy, published in India

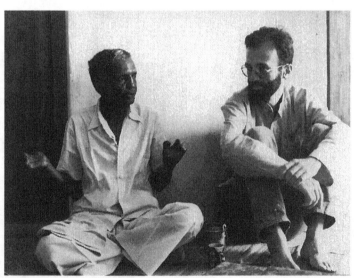

Madhava Rao (left) and Robert Helms (right) "Rao tells a story at our farewell dinner"

A Guinea Pig Among the Lepers
(Or, What I Did Once Between Drug Studies)
BY ROBERT HELMS, A.K.A. GUINEA PIG ZERO

A few years back, I had a string of paychecks that left me in good enough shape to take a nice, long vacation. My luck had run high through several months of hopping around the country to some not-too intrusive, low-end dosage, steady-stay drug studies that fattened up my wallet, didn't burn me out, and didn't let me spend much. I was in the mood to not be stabbed and drained for awhile, especially after being kept in-house on a boring diet for an entire month at the last place. On top of that, I had left my bag on a train and checked in without any of my own books, which put me at the mercy of one of those ratty little shelves that only a nurse manager would call a library, all romance novels and dog-eared copies of *In Search of Excellence*. I was saved by a copy of La Pierre's *City of Joy*, about slum life in Calcutta, India. I liked it so much that, despite its corny streak, I read it twice. Since I had already seen a lot of the U.S. travelling from study to study, I needed an exotic destination to keep me distracted for a few months, and the book helped me plan a trip to a region where food is spicy and television rare—India seemed to fit the bill nicely. Anyway, by the time my pockets were flush I had signed on as one of those worldly undergraduates doing a "semester abroad." Of course, I'm not after academic credentials: I had already earned my stripes as a practicing stick-pig and I just needed a sabbatical. I decided to do research on lepers.

I know what you're thinking: "Check out Mr. Goodie Two-shoes. He probably wants to be a priest!" Well, it's a fair assumption, but it turned out that the leprous life is in many ways like a guinea pig's sterile realm of vacuum

199

tubes and piss bottles, but transported to the fertile, cattle-filled streets of South Asia. A poor, leprosy-afflicted person can survive in Indian society by living under the wing of a charitable institution, wandering around begging, or both. In any case, the formula is that somebody takes pity on the sufferer and gives them what they need. In turn the leper does and says all the things that will help further this process.

By the way, it's politically incorrect to call them lepers; all the doctors and mucky-mucks say "leprosy victims." The people themselves laugh at this, showing you their fingerless hands saying, "Are you joking? Look at me! I'm a leper if there ever was one!" I think of this whenever a nurse calls me a "study subject" or a "volunteer." I bear no illusions about the economy of my flesh as I wander through this meat-rack of a world, and so I call myself a guinea pig.

I got my start by visiting a small leprosy asylum run by a richly endowed society of Mahatma Gandhi types. I met the staff and residents when the director graciously gave me a guided tour. The deformities include missing fingers, toes and entire limbs, as well as some very unfortunate collapsed noses. I volunteered to help change bandages on the ulcerous feet of folks who stopped in from the surrounding area. Madhava Rao, one of the resident leprosy victims, was a very interesting guy who spoke both English and Telugu, the region's language. He said he'd gladly work for me as a translator, and he could introduce me to more lepers than I could shake a stick at. We struck a deal that made sense for both of us and lasted for the next few months.

What's amazing about leprosy is the way it affects the nerves. I knew that it kills all peripheral sensation, but I was surprised to discover how far this actually goes. Rao himself once had to hop up on a gurney bed for treatment during one of the days I was working at an outpatient clinic. A winter virus had aggravated an ulcer on his big toe, and he needed to have the outermost digit amputated. This is actually how lepers lose their body parts—they don't simply fall off in the street like I used to think when I was a kid. The medical technician, who held no degree and was also mildly effected by the disease, opened up the wound and exposed the end of the toe-bone. Rao and I chatted during the procedure about a trip we were planning to a rural leper colony. As was the case in all of these treatments, no anesthesia was used. That was all well and good until the technician took out a pair of wire cutters and grabbed hold of Rao's little toe joint. I started fidgeting a little, glancing back and forth between Rao's foot and his face, then "SNAP!" and the piece of bone fell into a metal dish.

"Hold on a second!" I said. "Didn't you feel that? I mean, exactly what do you feel right now?"

The tech and his patient exchanged smiles. "Only a tingling sensation. Nothing like pain," Rao told me. "I swear, you could chop off one of my arms, and I'd hardly notice." He had adjusted to the numbness and seldom gave it a thought. Although I never discussed it with Rao, this outpatient clinic would become a sort of a gallery to me. I've browsed the Louvre and wandered the Prado, but no statue, no matter how clever the artist or how striking the material, can hold a candle to those wild sculptures of contorted feet. Muscles collapse where infected bones are removed, and huge calluses turn ankles, bridges, and soles into strange fists.

It would be easy to assume that the sexuality of lepers disappears along with their fingers and toes, but that's not the case, as the disease does not affect their genital nerves. This may help explain why they're able to maintain a sense of community after contracting the illness and not suffer

A Guinea Pig Among the Lepers (Or, What I Did Once Between Drug Studies)

a total loss of hope. At one colony we visited I learned how leprosy permanently separates these people from the rest of society and leaves them to create families from among their own. The disease drives all creeds and castes to leprosy communities, where one leper always seeks another as a mate and their children, unaffected by the sickness, will usually marry into other leper-families. Unlike the rest of Indian society, marriage across caste and religious lines are common among these people.

In the West economics will drive all creeds and castes into guinea pigging. Some of the oddest mixtures of people will be found together in the same study. The recession has thrown us off the gravy train and here we are, former accountants, bike messengers, factory hands, demobbed soldiers, and lots of college-aged economic refugees. It's not unusual for a hungry medical student to line up for a blood draw behind a guy who got his education at the state pen. But who will help us if we don't look after each other? We've got to milk the pharmaceutical cow with gentle fingers and watch each other's back, or else the thing will stomp us all into the dirt with its hooves.

And we deal with the same sorts of troubles as lepers do. I went to a colony that was run by Christian evangelists where I heard complaints about having to go to church and sing, but they couldn't drink, couldn't carouse with their lovers, and they had to finish every dried-up, cruddy meal without complaint, or else hit the road. Certain missionaries would wear out their employees at starvation wages, use the lepers as free labor and maintain the facilities only for show to secure donations from the West. Does this sound similar to any of research units you know?

Naturally, a measure of crap will sometimes roll from the lips of lepers, but for reasons of survival rather than greed. The typical leper will give outsiders a neatly prepared speech explaining why he begs, sort of like this:

> We come from decent but not wealthy families,
> where we're not welcome anymore because of our
> affliction. We never touch liquor. We can't find jobs,
> also for being lepers, and we'd gladly earn a living in
> any other way. We pray to lord Jesus and rely on his
> mercy. He is our only solace. We never beg on
> Sunday.

Since I was a devious outsider travelling with an insider dishing me all the dirt, I knew that there were some serious drinkers among the lepers, and that many of them were church-goers only the way some might belong to a political party—as long as it got them what they wanted or when there was little other choice. There was a correlation between staying on in the colony and converting to the management's creed.

Happily, I was to find that there were other colonies where the local religionists were honest and altruistic, but they could only afford to help with medicines and building supplies, which left the afflicted to rustle up their own food. To get money for food, the men at one community organize begging expeditions that go by rail through a circuit of nearby cities. For four days a week, they break up into groups of five or six and board trains leaving Anakapalle, in the state of Andhra Pradesh, about eighty miles from the coast. The trip takes them through Vizag, Rajamundry, Kakinada, Samalkot, then home again. They bum change from the passengers, then at the stations, and finally in the streets of the towns themselves. The conductors never charge them to ride because they are not even regarded as passengers; they're part of the railway culture, like the tea-sellers and the poor children who polish shoes. Besides, they don't occupy seats, and if they wanted it, they were technically entitled to a 75% discount. Trainmen would find it disgusting to stand there talking to them, and would prefer not to look in their direction. The money is divided equally among the members of each begging team, and the whole expedition rolls back into Anakapalle on Friday afternoon or evening.

This method does not bring in very much money and is extremely difficult during the hot season. I asked why they didn't go into the larger cities like Hyderabad or Madras where they'd find more tourists and traffic. They explained this would keep them from their families for too long, and some would be unable to go at all. Also, the farther they went from home, the more they would be trespassing on the turf of begging lepers from other areas. Without a sizeable group, I was told, they could not risk running into competition in the big cities. I told them that in my line of work we encounter similar problems and try to hang with a few friends whenever possible. The closer I get to New York or Chicago, the more touchy run-ins I seem to have with temperamental, street-talking city guys who leave me wondering, "How did I get here? All I want is a few hundred bucks so I can get back to the provinces."

Our minds really met when they told me about a big leprosy-relief honcho who once visited them and made speeches about setting them up in a candle-making business, giving their kids bicycle-rickshaws to earn a living, and maybe even throwing in a few chickens. They'd already had some sour experiences with promise-making politicians who posed for group photos and were never heard from again. Right after his big speech, the honcho asked them to assemble in front of the church for a picture, and the lepers did something quite unusual for such humble folk; they apologized for disappointing him, but they could not be photographed until after the promised benefits began to arrive. The official was insulted and severed all communications with this colony.

Unkept promises sounded all-too familiar. I told them about guinea pigs that I knew who went nearly to the end of a drug study only to be told they would receive no money because of a minor, house-rules transgression. Another trick is when a doctor sends a lab rat for a test because of some funny results during the study, then sends the lab rat a bill for the test which exceeds the money he got for doing the study! The value of the person's time was reduced to nothing and all the smiles and professional language had warped into lies. Just as the terms of charity are the bottom lines of business for a leper, a guinea pig must never let down his guard when discussing his body with a staffer. One might be chatting about baseball or joking about the day's news with a perfectly nice nurse, and in slips a careless comment relating to the drug study. The nurse wouldn't intend any harm, but would be duty-bound to record anything she learned about the patient's condition, and it could turn into a financial mess. Both lepers and guinea pigs have to exercise a little bit of business savvy.

As it drew time for me to fly home, I got together with some of my friends for some food, some arrack (a sort of bathtub gin made from palm fruit) and some serious lamplight storytelling. The guy with the fingers was buying. Several lepers told me how their families and castes had disowned them and how they learned to shun society out of shame for their deformities. I was listening as an objective outsider until one fellow related how difficult it was for him or any leper to receive the meager pension guaranteed them by the Indian government. He had once waited all day, only to be stonewalled by an "office peon," as clerks are actually called there. The leper said to the peon with absolute sincerity:

"You and I come from similar backgrounds, have the same level of education, and speak the same tongue. This sickness is so capricious that it doesn't strike one for reasons known to us, but for reasons known only to God. If I had not been effected by this disease as a boy, I would be a productive citizen today, and my life would be as yours is. Only for this do I find myself humbly approaching you, instead of addressing you as a perfect equal. Won't you give me your endorsement in this matter? It means a very great deal to me, whereas to you it makes no difference whatsoever. What prevents you from doing this small thing for me?"

He never received the pension.

One woman told of the agony that she suffered when given the multi-drug therapy (a combination of three medicines that cures leprosy at early stages and can arrest the disease at any stage). She was given the wrong dosages by a less than excellent physician—it was worse than anything leprosy had done to her, she said, and it lead to her present sickliness. I had already learned that these mishaps were known to happen. I once saw a man who had been blinded by a similar multi-drug therapy miscalculation; but I was also once introduced to a beautiful, bright-eyed eleven-year old girl who had been completely cured by the same process (correctly administered, of course). The woman telling me her story stressed how grateful people should be that I was risking my life to eliminate diseases from the world. I politely thanked her.

When with these people, I discovered other ways in which the leper social life resonates with the guinea pig existence, namely in how they're perceived. Even though my relatively comfortable experience is nowhere comparable to the poverty and disability of these people, they remained wide-eyed and nodding while Rao translated what I was saying about the social aspects of being a guinea pig. We guinea pigs are no strangers to professional life, and we are often more qualified in our respective fields than the nurses are in theirs. Yet it's not uncommon to be treated like we're naughty children who need to be locked in, threatened and continually observed before we can be relied upon to pee in a bottle and roll up our sleeves.

There's some kind of stigma in this line of work that echoes the social shunning lepers deal with, albeit nowhere near the severity. Once I was having lunch with my girlfriend and her mom, and a hard look was shot my way when I started to talk about a study I had just completed. My girlfriend later told me that it was better not to discuss my work because the old lady would misinterpret it, thinking I was some kind of derelict selling plasma for five bucks a pint. In order to preserve the peace, she'd just rather not deal with it. Here I was, more clean-cut and drug-free than the next fifty people she's likely to meet, doing an entirely legal, 99% safe activity to earn money. Furthermore, I'm operating independently and retain my mind and creative energy while renting my body to science brings home some cash. For all that, my line of work is relegated to something like pushing dope in front of a school or pimping women on some street corner.

When pharmacologists, nurses and medical technologists go out with their mates, do they conceal the exact nature of their work? Do they say "I'm in a surgical unit" or "I have a desk job?" Of course they don't, and since their work is dependent upon me and happens inside my squeaky-clean body, my character is no more questionable than theirs. Humanity being such an ignorant thing, though, guinea pigs will never eliminate this stigma from social life. There's no moral logic to it, so it must be a money thing; since the staffer has more cash in the bank than I do, certain people with office peon mentalities use this easy excuse to sneer.

As I said goodbye to my friends in India, they kept telling me to "watch out for those doctors" and called upon God to watch over me. I thanked them for helping me to understand myself by sharing their stories, and I urged them to put their heads together for a decisive victory over the peons. I knew then why outcasts must form associations and rely upon each other if they want any chance of squeezing a decent life out of this world.

A Thin Man's Tale
BY ROBERT HELMS

For human guinea pigs, fasting and observing strict dietary restrictions are basic professional responsibilities. We fast the night before a screening date, and if we cheat, our blood sugar levels will be too high to qualify. A poppyseed bagel the day prior to a drug screen can come up positive for recreational opiates. In many studies there is an eight-hour fasting period after dosing time so the drug can be more carefully tracked through the blood stream. Another common thing is to eat only what they give you, all of what they give you, and sometimes exactly in the half-hour time slot starting when they put the tray in front of you.

A typical protocol will say an eligible volunteer must be *within 10% of his or her ideal weight.* This is determined by measuring the width of your elbow joint with a calliper to get your frame size, then checking on a chart to see how much space you should take up. If you're skinny, you'd better not be 'big boned,' because if you are, you have no right to be so thin, and you won't qualify. Likewise, if you're short and fat or tall and skinny, forget it. I have just enough meat on me to not look funny, so I always get through this particular hurdle.

One of my drug studies was at the Clinical Pharmacology Unit in Ben Tucker Memorial. This unit was owned by the hospital until it was bought by an independent firm that underbids competition for experiment contracts. They hire their own non-union staff, cater their own meals and buy their own supplies. It's been this way ever since a Kuwaiti sheikh bought up every hospital in town and then started trimming the fat from his empire. I only know this because my two sisters are nurses and they always go on about how it's all going to the dogs.

Science is just a job for these health care professionals, and their interest is in doing the job as cheaply as possible. This is most apparent at meal times. In this experiment at Tucker Hospital only meat eaters like myself were allowed into the study. A vegetarian guy I used to chat with had lied to get in and tried to eat as little meat as possible, so he'd sneak me his Salisbury steak and I'd toss him a wad of macaroni. Once a nurse spotted us and threatened to dock our pay if we did it again. She watched us like a hawk after that.

We were galled when, because of complaints, the staff switched to a different (and much better) caterer in the middle of our study, yet every group of volunteers had to stay on their own diet until a study was complete to preserve the consistency of their data. Since our study had begun several months earlier, we had to stay on our current diets. This wouldn't have been so bad except for newer studies that began with guinea pigs who got better food from the new caterer.

The dining room where we ate became more crowded one day after a nurse made a new dinner announcement: "Pfizer guys, time to eat!" Us guinea pigs were colorcoded in hospital scrubs according to their studies, and about a dozen new guys in blue pajamas hurried in to open the Styrofoam trays that had been laid out at certain tables. This was their first meal in the unit. My vegetarian buddy, wearing bright orange pajamas like mine, waved to a guy in blue he knew who was settling down a few feet away from us. "Nice blues," he said. "Yeah, thanks. I see they gave you the orange, so if you escape, they can spot you real easy. They make the chain gang wear the same color," his friend quipped.

"Is it true they've got gun towers on the roof here?" I asked.

"Hey, you never know," Blue said with a smile. "When are you guys getting out?"

"Tomorrow morning, between nine and eleven," said veggie Orange. "They told us it should go quickly but they don't want to promise... Oh, my God, what's this?"

The man in blue pajamas had broken the flow of ideas with a harsh physical maneuver: he had opened the top of his food tray. Our eyes fixed on the lively colors of a square of lasagna; a heavy slice of apple pie with big, clumsy crumbs and raisins peeking out from its cinnamon-laden guts with a dollop of whipped cream lying across its top; a cluster of steamy, peppered chicken slices that gleamed with moisture; and finally some thickly buttered snow peas that held themselves with a firmness that disclosed in no uncertain terms that they had been living, growing vegetables mere hours before offering themselves up to be devoured.

We then turned our heads back to the barren fare we'd been picking at. The macaroni shells took up most of each tray and wore just enough grease to help them fall away from each other. When eaten, these cheeseless things resisted the teeth as if the pasta were pulled from the pot too soon. The stuff had merely been softened enough to digest without major gastric distress, and with none of the flavor one would find in imported or even regular name brand macaroni. Another pocket of the tray held spinach from a can, a food familiar enough to forego description. Lastly, the meat loaf represented both the animal and vegetable kingdoms in such a way as to evade any ingredient descriptions like beef or rice. This was 'meat product,' with some gravy.

We in the orange pajamas looked at our plates, and our stomachs spoke together, saying that they didn't like being treated this way. A young nurse kept eyeing us from nearby as she locked the stainless steel refrigerators while sipping her cup of normal, caffeinated coffee. I always miss the coffee. Our noses were brought back to the other table by the wonderful smells.

"Relax, man," said the blue guinea pig as he cut into the lasagna with the side of his fork, "eighteen more hours and you'll be out there having fun with your paycheck— what are you doing, the blood thinner? seventeen hundred?—and I'll be in here with the needles and the TV set. What's the first thing you're going to eat?"

"Right," I said, "best to think about the real world. First off I'll be getting a double espresso, then I think I'll get lunch at one of those Ethiopian places near the university. The *injera* really fills you all the way up, and the spices are pretty special. Ever tried it?"

Blue nodded that he had, but I sensed he had no immediate need to remember. Another guy became interested and said he should check out East African cuisine sometime soon. While everyone ate the conversation wandered from one exotic eatery to another. As we walked our trash to the garbage can, I mused about being in a real restaurant and finishing up with a nice cigar. Dining companions of both colors shot me a look, then discreetly glanced in the direction of the nurse. She hadn't heard the remark.

"Careful," said Orange when we got to the TV room. "A friend of mine slipped up once when being interviewed by a rookie doctor. She asked if he was a smoker, and of course my man says 'No,' but then he goes, 'I did smoke a cigar a few weeks ago after I ate,' and she cut the dude right out of the study. He was out nine hundred bucks on one lousy cigar. That's *nine beans!*"

Since our group had just finished its dreary meal, almost every guinea pig in the TV room was lean and young and in orange like myself. There were also a few guys in green who were trying out a new antidepressant, but they simply stared at the monitor with their usual serene expressions. Barely a word had passed between them since I was admitted a week earlier. 'Brain sluts' are pretty disgusting, when you stop to think about it, becoming retarded for money like that.

We arrived in the middle of the six o'clock news. "They stuff their faces for science! Chomping down ten thousand calories a day and getting paid to do it in a new obesity study at Tucker Hospital, when we come right back!" The newswoman announced this like a bad actress trying to generate an amazed voice. The chubby face of a blond woman shovelling ravioli into her mouth briefly flashed on the screen. Then we caught a close-up of a man's bearded face consuming some sort of milk shake, then wiping his mouth with a tired expression.

A long "whooaa!" came from the ten or twelve articulate viewers while the boys in green raised their eyebrows and smiled a bit more widely, looking around at their excited neighbors. As the commercials rattled by the rest of us traded exclamations of disbelief.

"Here I am starving half the time and eating dog food the other half, and they're getting paid to pig out? It's too much," I said.

"And in the same building, no less," another guy remarked. "Maybe there's more to this study than they told us. Maybe they're studying the extent to which people will tolerate lousy food, and we're really all getting a placebo in the arm."

The news program came back on the air and the reporter spoke as a long table filled with food appeared on the screen:

"Breakfast consisted of two sausage sandwiches with eggs, hotcakes with butter and syrup, and several servings of hash browns. That was for starters. As the day waddled on, the ten volunteers in this scientific experiment also packed away chicken, jumbo-sized cheeseburgers, french fries, two pints of ice cream and eight ounces of cashews, for a whopping total of 10,000 calories."

We were silent as our sullen faces fixed on the monitor. "The experiment is not to find out who's the biggest pig," the voice continued, "but rather to study a hormone called leptin (the Greek word for thin), which is thought to be an important regulator of body fat." The scene broke to show a doctor measuring the fat on a woman's arm with a skin-fold calliper. "They're making sure *she's* fat—but we had to prove *we're* skinny!" yelled a thin man. "And they make us get skinnier!" shouted another. The news person went on about how mice lost weight when injected with the new hormone, how a third of the U.S. population is obese, how chunkiness is getting more common, and how they needed more time to figure out *leptin* and how it could be profitable. The din remained fairly loud as the camera went from scientists in white to white rats and back to scientists.

"Hey, yo! Look! Check it out!" one of my orange buddies shouted from the window. "There she is! That's them!" The rest of us were momentarily confused and not happy to be distracted from the stimulating program, but he had spotted the face-stuffer study through a window three floors below us and across a wide courtyard. "I thought they looked familiar," he continued. "Let me get my specs." He rushed out to his bedroom and came back with a small pair of opera glasses. Guinea pigs occasionally include these in their personal travel kit in case there's a dormitory full of cute nurses nearby, or just to people-watch the sidewalks below.

We formed a group beside the window, our attention split between the fish tank TV screen with its talking heads and the window some fifty yards off. The guys started passing the glasses around, trying to determine what was on the dining table in that happier place, so close yet so far away. "I see french fries... I think that's spaghetti... What's the guy eating? Pancakes? No, waffles. They're giving them waffles!" When my turn came, I watched the awful spectacle of a lady in an easy chair biting into a big, sloppy sandwich I couldn't help but recognize. "Hogg's Deli. She's eating a spicy chicken hog."

This meant the researchers were ordering in food from around the neighborhood. One of my absolute favorite lunch items in the world is at Hogg's. They carve out the inside of a loaf of home-made bread that's still slightly moist from the steam table, stuff it with a delicious assortment of peppered chicken, blue cheese dressing and other salad ingredients, then serve it with some long, roasted peppers.

All of the guys who lived in the area knew what a spicy chicken hog was. We were getting really excited. One guy pressed his hands to his temples, saying, "Shit. Oh, shit." The news person was still speaking: "Dr. Wendy Thayer, Director of Clinical Research, says that she's been very discreet about the study, which pays its subjects $250 per day; 'We were afraid that we'd be overwhelmed with calls from people who'd want to participate.'"

Upon hearing this, everyone got up, yelling at the top of their lungs and slamming their fists down on the furniture. The TV room door was open the whole time, so the sounds were easily heard from nursing station down the hall. A narrow-minded and unpopular nurse came in. She was a no-nonsense school-marmish pain in the ass that couldn't find your vein with an anatomy map. Most of the guys in this study were a dozen years her senior and several were far more educated. For the most part we either ignored her or tried to limit our contact with her.

"OK guys, you know the rules," she proclaimed. "I'm gonna start docking paychecks if you don't quiet down!"

Everyone turned and faced her at the same moment. The whole group was standing. For a few seconds everyone was silent and stared straight into her face. The only sounds were chairs being pushed against tables, a book falling to the floor, and some long, disgusted groans coming from the hollows of our stomachs. The nurse's face lost its air of authority as her expression turned to actual fear, I suppose from all the bodies and raw displeasure aimed at her. She stepped backward, bumping into the doorframe, saying "Umm, umm…"

I could not control the peal of laughter that forced its way from my lungs. I felt like someone was holding me down tickling me and I was trying to wiggle free. I wanted to stop laughing, but it kept getting worse after each pause for breath. I wanted to leave the room, but the nurse was standing in the doorway and I didn't want to give the impression that I was advancing on her. I felt someone slap me on the back, and all at once everyone in orange pajamas burst out laughing in a single roar; even the brain sluts in green added some feeble nodding to their vapid smiles. The unhappy woman took off down the hall, and opinions differ as to whether she cried or not—we couldn't be sure.

In the end she half-heartedly tried to fine each of us twenty-five bucks, but we were able to talk the more mature director out of it. After leaving with our pay envelopes, we walked down to the face-stuffers' ward to ask questions and sign up, but somehow they were expecting us and kept refusing to buzz us in. I wandered off with two Belgian guinea pigs to introduce them to spicy chicken hogs, and they gave me the rundown on lab ratting in their country. They told me that when they go home to Brussels and talk about our horrible drug study food, nobody ever believes them. Finally we said goodbye, and I went to visit my bank.

The Enema

BY OCTAVE MIRBEAU

translated by Robert Helms

The story first appeared under the title "En Viager" in Le
Journal *in Paris, August 12, 1894.*

At the end of fifteen years of pharmaceutical practice,
Monsieur Latête, a pharmacist first class, ex-intern of the
hospitals of Toulouse, laureate of many academies and
provincial learned societies, with diverse specialties, a gold
medal, et cetera, perceived that counting solely on his
earnings from his job he would never quite reach the point
where he could dote adequately upon his daughters. He
had five of them, and as a good father to his family, jeal-
ous for the happiness of his children, it was his ambition
to set them up beautifully. Besides, his was a legitimate
ambition because M. Latête was considered a big shot in
the town. He was deputy mayor; a councilor of the
arrondissement; the president of the independent voters'
committee; the intimate friend of an opportunistic deputy
(by whom he was assured the election); founder of the
region's mutual society of cyclists; and Secretary-Treasurer
of the SouthWestern Archaeologists' Group. He was also
decorated by Agricole, an officer of the Academy, and had
been appointed to the highest functions and given the
most direct honors. It goes without saying that he was
honest and a partisan of all authorities—one who respected all laws and defended all established institutions.

He was, in our view, a model citizen, but his overhead
was heavy: the political dinner parties, his wife's wardrobe,
the high-class education he wanted for his daughters—all
of this cost him plenty. The pharmacy yielded a good
return, 100%, just as with all pharmacies, but by the end

of the year M. Latête didn't succeed in setting aside all the money he wished to have. It's true that he had been unlucky in various extra-professional enterprises, that he had suffered considerable losses speculating in Turkey and Panama, and that he was a silent partner in some plaster kilns and a parcel delivery service that hadn't turned out well. "Bah!" he said to himself, "One day I'll find something reliable." Taking a cue from some of his colleagues, he dreamed of discovering marvelous syrups and magic lozenges, but then he discovered something better to sell.

There was a nice old guy who often came to his store, an unmarried man with no direct heirs who constantly complained about managing his property. M. Latête knew at a glance that this was a sick man with a feeble character who wanted to feel better. One day the pharmacist asked the man, "Why don't you put your fortune into a lifetime annuity? You'll double your income, and you won't have any worries."

"An annuity!" the old guy exclaimed, "Oh, thanks a lot, but no thanks. I wouldn't sleep so well. One never knows who's going to get the fortune. I wouldn't be comfortable, I'm afraid. No, no. There are so many murderers about these days—and so many anarchists!"

"Probably," the pharmacist concurred, "and I wouldn't advise you to do business with the first guy that comes along! The Devil knows it's delicate, handling these things. But you'll find someone safe, a serious man, thank you, a regular guy; there's bound to be one around here somewhere, thank God, what with all the new laws. Hey, this will relieve you beautifully! Beyond all the liabilities, temptations, and covetousness that surround you, you'll have absolute liberty and complete tranquillity—a real paradise. You'll finally be able to enjoy life! And besides that, don't you know, this way a sou is worth two sous, a franc's worth two francs, and a thousand francs, two thousand. Ha, ha! And needless to say, you're still as sturdy as an oak!"

"Me?" The old guy interjected piteously. "But I'm sick—awfully sick! I don't sleep, I don't eat..."

"—Tut, tut, tut!" M. Latête replied, shrugging his shoulders. "Is it the doctors who tell you such nonsense? Of course, it's their job! But I, who am also a doctor; I who can tell what people have in their stomachs at a glance; indeed, I tell you that you carry yourself admirably. Oh, I'd tell those doctors to go take a hike!" He then declared with an air of regret, "Look, if I were like you and didn't have a family to get started in life, and if I were in such robust health as yourself, I'd have long since put my fortune into an annuity!"

The old guy exclaimed, "You? M. Latête!"

"Yes, me! That's right, I guarantee you that. And you know what else I'll tell you? I'll take your fortune myself, at ten-percent interest. It's foolish, I know, but what can it do to me? I'm like you; I love to render service. I don't suppose you're afraid of me, now, are you?"

"You, M. Latête? Well, how about that!" The old fellow's face first twisted into strange grimaces, then into a most lively expression of surprise, then delight. "Well," he repeated, "how about that!"

The next day M. Latête paid a visit to the old fellow's doctor. He wanted to know certain bits of confidential information about the old man. The physician instantly pleaded professional secrecy.

"Oh, well," M. Latête argued, "between doctor and pharmacist there is no question of such confidentiality. Besides, the fellow's an old relation of mine, whom I love very, very much. I'm really worried about his health. He treats himself like shit. He has crazy spells that could become dangerous. Someone has to keep an eye on him. Look, just between me and you, a respected physician, what do you think?"

"All right then, just between us," the doctor said in a tone of confidence, "I believe that the old guy has a bad stone in his belly. My God, with some care and inflexible discipline, he could go on like this for some years more, but, above all, no dissipation! He has this crazy idea, against which I have all the difficulty in the world protecting him. He wants to give himself an enema—he doesn't enjoy being sick like that. But an enema could be fatal to him. There's been every reason to fear an intestinal hemorrhage, and hell, that'll be the end of him!"

For some time they chatted about medicine, about their affection for the old guy, they discussed certain possibilities, and finally they came to the conclusion that the man should undergo a moderate treatment.

"Perfectly so!" the pharmacist summed up, proudly embellishing with the noblest analogies. "His stomach deserves freedom, but not license!"

"Just as in politics, my dear sir," the doctor concluded, "all organisms resemble each other. They function by the same needs and they're damaged by the same causes. It ought to work in medicine the same way as in sociology."

"The stomach is funny," remarked the honorable pharmacist, "when it comes to taking a holiday."

The annuity deal was closed that same evening. The following week, the document to allow the pharmacist was irrevocably signed, registered in accordance with all the legal requirements, and entered in among the number of other finalized affidavits. At the same time as fortune went out through the front door of the good fellow's house, death was coming in through the back.

Three days later the old guy, who never left the pharmacy any more, complained to M. Latête: "It won't go away!" he moaned, "I don't know what it is that I have. My head is spinning, I feel all dizzy, my stomach feels weird, and my guts are going crazy! It won't go away!"

"It's the springtime!" the good pharmacist pronounced categorically. "Spring brings on these same effects for me, too. There's no reason to worry. A little enema and it'll all be taken care of. I gave myself an enema yesterday, and you ought to do it tomorrow!"

The old guy became scared. "An enema! That's what I've been telling you! But I'm specifically forbidden to do it!"

M. Latête laughed. "Of course! Those doctors don't go for the real remedies. They're just dragging things out—it's quite understandable. But in the end it's your own business, so you can do whatever you want!"

"Seriously," the old guy insisted, "do you think so?"

"A vial of German spirits, a glass of wine, all in ten minutes," M. Latête confirmed. "There you go. That's what I take. And the next day? Fresh as a daisy, happy as a bird, strong as a Turk."

"Well, good then—give me one! After all, those doctors sure do as they please for themselves!" He took the vial away with him.

When the old man had left, M. Latte joyously rubbed his hands together and, at the thought of the news that he could not fail to receive the next morning, he murmured mischievously, "A legal enema!"

The Mouse & Sammy Snake

BY ROBERT HELMS

Way, way back in the mid-1950's, when most of us were not even a twinkle in our daddy's eye, there were certain persons at Duke University who knew about Sammy Snake.

Harriet was a very smart gal, as was everyone at Durham, North Carolina's elite college. She was working her way through her undergraduate studies as a laboratory assistant. However, like most very bright people, Harriet did not take well to being told what she could and could not do. At times this made her life at Duke rather irritating. There were strict curfews, gender segregation and all sorts of rules of conduct that were heavily enforced. Adding insult to injury were the rules forbidding any pets from being kept in the dormitories.

"How about that," said the young woman, "It's like we're children, like we can't look after a cat or a little dog."

She carefully looked over her handbook during breakfast one morning. After the general statement against animals, there were specific examples listed so that clever scofflaws could not meander through the rules with some critter not mentioned. Harriet wished to do just that, so she traced her fingers down the row, past dogs, cats, guppies, goats, parrots, canaries, and so forth.

"How about that," said the young scholar, "the university seems to have no problem with boa constrictors."

Soon Harriet had set up her small dormitory room with a large terrarium. Inside there were a few rocks, a 9-foot long, thick-bodied, very hungry boa, and not much else. The new resident was given the name Sammy Snake and soon he became a source of evening entertainment for his owner and her circle of friends.

Every few weeks, as the petite young lady finished her work at the laboratory, she would reach down into the holding tank for mice after they had completed their roles in some experiment. Then she would snatch a white mouse in her hand and deftly hide it in the pocket of her plaid cotton dress, close the button on the pocket and walk home to the dorm. These little animals were killed as a matter of policy and not sold to pet stores or given away as pets. Lab animals, like meat-industry livestock, spend their whole existence under a death sentence, and when they have served their purpose they are destroyed.

On the way out of the lab Harriet would often invite a friend or two over for a cup of tea, and as they sipped and chatted a little white mouse would be placed inside the terrarium with old Sammy. Instead of being drowned and thrown into the college incinerator, the mouse would be spotted by the enormous reptile, then swallowed whole and dissolved in Sammy's stomach. Everyone except the mouse benefited in this new meal plan: science marched on, Sammy had his lunch, Harriet's room became the place to gossip for a discreet few, and the lab administrators lost nothing in the bargain.

Some months passed, as Harriet continued her studies and the great snake gobbled his mice. Then one morning Harriet emerged from the dorm with a long face and sad, red eyes. Her schoolmate Jan spotted her in the library, a tall, strapping fellow who divided his time between botany, Bach and football. As they crossed paths Jan quietly approached Harriet and asked what was the matter.

"Sammy Snake is dead," she whimpered, "and you will never believe what killed him! I brought him a mouse last night, just as I always do, and a few minutes later it was all over. The mouse killed him!"

"Huh?" Jan asked, flabbergasted. "That can't be. Let's go have a look."

They hurried over to Harriet's room, picking up a few other friends along the way. Inside the glass walls of the long terrarium a little white mouse sat atop the great serpent, calmly nibbling at a small wound at the nape of Sammy's neck.

Indeed, Sammy Snake was no more. His spine had been severed: The mouse had jumped to avoid Sammy's deadly jaws, landed on his back and had bitten into a certain vulnerable spot along Sammy's spinal column. The diner and his lunch had switched places.

"Well, I'll be damned," said Jan when all the humans had finished gasping, "that little mouse must have a bit of mongoose in him. I wonder if he got this way from the experimental drug they gave him at the lab."

The teenagers were not in a position to investigate the scientific aspects of this wondrous event. Harriet would be severely disciplined for having the boa inside the dorm, and diverting mice from one death chamber to another would only make matters worse. The only thing to do was to stuff the lifeless body of Sammy Snake in a shopping bag, take him into town, and discreetly drop him in a municipal trash can when no one was looking. She did all this with sad determination and a friend making sure that the coast was clear.

When she returned home that evening Harriet walked slowly over to the terrarium and gazed into the eyes of the little white mouse. She suddenly felt respect and admiration for it, and found herself wondering whether it was male or female. This amazing creature had gone from anonymous experimental material to Tuesday's lunch to conquering hero, all by its own bravery and cunning.

"Well," Harriet sighed, "I guess I'll have to give you a name." She cleaned out the droppings of the unfortunate boa and foraged around for some crackers and celery for her valiant new pet to eat. After a little while she carefully reached in and lifted the mouse's tail, then gently and respectfully set it back down.

"It figures you'd be a girl. I'll name you Murida Constrictica—the girlmouse who conquered the boa."

Murida lived about another two years, and she had all the space she knew what to do with in that huge terrarium. Her proud owner brought her toys and wheels to play with and fussed and bragged about Murida to her friends. Harriet graduated and went off to who knows where and lost touch with Jan, who now spends some six hours each day at the piano, who still relishes the Bach, and who passed this true tale of heroism on to *Guinea Pig Zero*.

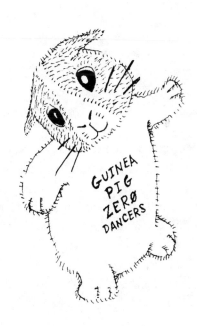

GUINEA PIG ZERØ DANCERS

Dialing For Disaster: A Guinea Pig Tale, Based on Real Rumors
BY ROBERT HELMS

Not so long ago, in a research unit in the U.S. there was a group of guinea pigs who spent a lot of time on the public pay phones. Naturally this created a problem of large phone bills. According to a recent scoop, a few of them were doing some kind of "phone phreaking," to avoid paying for the calls. Heaven knows that our responsibilities can take us far from home, and when we find ourselves cooped up in a hospital ward for the fifteenth or twentieth day, all for the good of humanity, we just might go to desperate extremes in order to hear the voice of a love one. Supposedly, one of these good men had a modified dialer which imitated the beeps that are normally made by quarters as they fell into the telephone.

A problem arose when an operator figured out what they were up to and then figured out what kind of place the pay phone was located in. There are special teams of technicians now, who have joined forces with the Federal Communications Commission (FCC), and these teams travel around in trucks trying to catch people in the act of making the recorded voice stop saying "please deposit," and say "thank you" instead. The drug study gave them a perfect environment for easy arrests. Normally, they will have a hard time getting to the telephone before the person finishes the trick call, and there will be too much anonymous confusion on a street, in a train station, or at a shopping mall. This time, however, they had a whole slew of guys who weren't going anywhere, all saving quarters in the same way.

The day nurses were busy preparing for the last big blood draw of a long and important clinical trial. Three of them hurried from bed to bed, carefully laying out an absorbant pad by each, and on it five vacuum tubes, a plastic syringe, a butterfly tube, a rubber tourniquet, a small gauze pad, and, of course, a band-aid with Disney characters on it—even though most of the guys would decline to use them on their track marks. This was a platelet aggregation check, to be followed by the ever-popular *bleeding time*. The investigational drug was a blood thinner, and everyone was being dosed at various levels until they discovered the point at which the stuff would make you a hemophiliac. Some of the bleeding times coincided exactly with the blood draws, so that there would be a nurse on each arm, one very jolly with vampire jokes, counting the seconds before a small stab wound would stop producing little drops of blood, and the other just sucking the stuff up into tubes. They'd make the guys lie still in bed for half an hour before each one of these routines, as though wanting them to be in a state of grace before the ordeal. Warm rods of sun light reached across a row of freshly made beds to illuminate the crisp spine of Bergson's *Creative Evolution* that lay on an end-table shelf under a digital blood pressure machine.

The FCC attack squad had monitored the phones for days, and the time had come for them to close in on their game. They calmly put down their pornographic magazines, finished their donuts and drove to the research unit. Once they arrived, all six of them stormed in, rupturing the serene, scientific atmosphere with the sounds of their heavy boots. Some had 9mm pistols strapped to their hips, while others were armed with tool belts and those little phone-testing hand sets. Racks filled with empty test tubes rattled, and the eyes of a lab technician opened wide behind her mask and eye-shield as a vial of fresh urine fell from her gloved hand and splashed on the counter before her. Two young women in the waiting room on their first screening visits froze in their chairs, each clutching a clipboard with both hands.

The charge nurse was about to announce to the volunteers that they should finish their phone calls and lie down in bed, but she never got the first word out of her mouth. She walked out of the bedroom area and stepped into the recreation room, where three men were deeply involved in conversations on the pay phones with their feet propped up on chairs and window sills. As she emerged through the doorway, one of the feds, with a blonde crew cut, dark glasses, and a brown bomber jacket, was moving along the hall at such a speed that when he collided with the petite woman she went tumbling spread-eagle onto the extra bed that was kept in the corner for new recruits and the night shift to sleep on. Her bare shins and big sneakers stuck straight up in the air as her loose scrubs slid down to her knees, and, naturally, she started to scream.

The bulls charged across the room toward the bank of phones. A few guys were lounging on couches with big glasses of water watching a video of "The Sound of Music," and had just gotten to the part where some Gestapo agents arrive to cross-examine Julie Andrews in her classroom, but these couch potatoes never heard the dialogue, having turned their startled faces elsewhere.

A large hand closed around a young man's narrow wrist, just where a wide sheet of clear tape held the Teflon catheter in his vein, and where lazy blobs of saline solution and diluted blood traded places in the little tube. The other two callers began to stand and say "Wha..." and were pushed back down again by federal hands. The one in the bomber jacket yelled "Police! Hand over the devices!" He then muscled a guinea pig away from the phone, leaving the receiver dangling by its cord, and a tiny voice calling, "Daddy! Daddy!"

Just as the intruders were about to achieve total control over the bodies of their prey, one of the callers made a sudden movement with his free hand. A palm-sized black plastic box emerged from his nimble fingers, its altitude increasing as it glanced off the recycling bin marked "aluminum," then spinning in the air as it touched the tiny black & white TV monitor surveying the elevators outside the unit, and then tracing a smooth, straight line along the counter of the nurses' station, hitting a pen-light bearing the trendy slogan of a newly marketed antidepressant and leaving it spinning rapidly on the peach-colored formica surface as it flew off the other end and over a carpeted aisle where the door of the volunteers' bathroom was swinging open, allowing the little box to dive gracefully into the toilet bowl, where an honest research subject had just left a hard-earned crap. It ended its fateful journey with a "plop." From the recreation room, a leg, wearing rolled-up sweat pants and a green terry-cloth hospital bootie, was seen reaching for the flusher from behind the door. A cheer went up from the guinea pigs as the gurgling suction was heard.

Mid-way through the flight of the tiny box the bulls had begun pursuing it. During those precious seconds when the box whirled round and round in the filthy water, they were stomping back through the long room, and one phone-tech guy entered and plunged his arm into the bowl as its recent user was washing his hands. The arm re-emerged bearing no electronic device, but just a bit of mud instead.

The charge nurse was back on her feet and demanding answers, and the FCC men were showing their badges, which she didn't care to see. This lady had spent some years on duty in a busy city Emergency Room and in Psychiatric Intensive Care before taking her present position in order to see more of her family. Muscles and guns simply did not impress her. As she stared into the squinting, ignorant eyes of the wearer of the bomber jacket, she seemed to grow in physical size as her steady, authoritative voice increased in volume, soon dominating all the other sounds in the room.

"State your business."

"FCC, Ma'am. Sorry for the disturbance but..."

"You're in a hospital. You have assaulted the staff and the patients. You'd better have reasons for doing this. Also, you will be held responsible for any damage you do to our research."

"Police business, Ma'am, we have reason to believe that.."

"Get to the point," the nurse interrupted, "Is this a drug bust? Well, what?"

The agents all glanced at each other. Three were coming from the bank of phones, where they had searched the three guys whose calls were interrupted. They were shaking their heads in disappointment. The other came from the bathroom wiping off his fingers with a brown paper towel, "Nothing either," he said.

A tall guinea pig named Hank, with thick glasses and long blond curls, emerged from the bedroom. He had been sleeping off a long morning of making calls and reading the *Racing Form* and *The Wall Street Journal*, which had arrived for him that morning by messenger. The other volunteers looked at him with an expectant smile. The nurse found herself distracted by his entry, wondering whether all the confusion was some how connected to him. She paused for a moment, while he began to speak.

"This, my friends, was not mentioned in the protocol," he began, "and therefore, it will need to be explained."

The federal agent started his explanation haltingly: "Illegally modified dialers have been in use here, and—"

"Rubbish!" yelled Hank, "If that's true, then either arrest somebody, or shut up and get out. We work for a living!"

"Stay out of it, Hank," the nurse cut in firmly, wishing to remain in control. Then she turned again to the goons. "I want to know your names, then out you go. You've already screwed up the study, and someone's going to pay for it."

Just then the doors opened at both ends of the unit, and twelve large men entered smoothly, all of them exactly the same height and just able to walk through the doorways without ducking down. Other features were strikingly similar as well, like the skin tone, eye color, and weight, but these similarities were not easily observed. Each was wearing a different outfit, hair color and style, and a few wore eyeglasses. They stepped two by two alongside each of the intruders, and stared down into their now-timid faces. All of the guinea pigs were on their feet, some standing on chairs to see over the crowded room to where the main players were facing each other down. The men now entering were known to a few of the volunteers, having appeared once or twice when a fight erupted between two guys, or when a fellow had started shrieking at a nurse for gouging him during a blood draw. At other times these mooses might be seen reading a newspaper in the lobby, trimming the bushes in a courtyard, or biting a sandwich in the lunchroom, but never speaking to anyone, and never all together like this in one room.

The door at the far end of the scene offered one last form. A tall, slender woman in a scarlet jacket and a long, black cotton skirt walked with unhurried steps toward the cluster of bodies, which parted gently, allowing her to pass. Her thick auburn hair wandered in the most graceful curls from her pale forehead to her cheeks, ever so soft-looking, down along the smooth, gentle lines of her neck, then splashing past her shoulders and down to the small of her back. A single lock, however, fell forward onto the lapel of her jacket, its lazy spiral swaying as she moved, leading the eye to the neckline of her buttoned shirt, whose delicate, printed roses tumbled dizzily around the proud curvatures of her breasts. As this dreamy image glided past her silent observers, leaving in her wake the faint scent of lilac perfume, their wet eyes fixed upon the lush movement of her buttocks as they rocked softly beneath the thin cotton. Less clearly defined were the shapes of her elegant thighs and knees, reaching down still farther to the red embroidered hem of her skirt as it danced against the backs of her pale calves. From there, two fine ankles were exposed to view, one carrying a thin golden chain; the other the tattooed design of an iris. On her feet were soft sandals of black leather, and red paint tickled on her toenails. As she reached the spot where the nurse and the G-men were standing, a ray of sunlight reached between the shoulders of two of the silent giants as between the trees of an ancient forest, to illuminate her head and chest, making her hair glow suddenly red and her wide green eyes sparkle in their full glory. As she came to a halt, her soft parts jiggled ever so slightly.

The charge nurse, like the volunteers, knew this person well but had never seen her in civilian clothes. She was just as taken back as they were by the power the garments added to her already formidable appearance. Although guinea pigs would speculate in quiet terms about whether she was married, or various stories they'd heard about her being a champion swimmer or an accomplished violinist, without exception they revered her and were quiet and respectful in her presence. If she happened to make an adverse decision that excluded a guy from a study for high bilirubin or low sugar, he would calmly agree that she knew best instead of whining for the blood work to be repeated. A certain fellow made a vulgar remark about her over lunch once, and then failed to appear for check-in time at the next leg of the study. That was it: no one saw him or spoke of him again. He had been made ineligible for the study and terribly unwelcome by his former colleagues.

The nurse cleared her throat, then said, "Hello, Doctor Butters."

The doctor's voice needed no loudness to be heard in the silence that awaited it. "You people have made a great mistake," she said to the outsiders, "in stepping between me and my patients. My friends will remove you from the building."

One of the FCC agents made a last attempt to assert himself. "Uh, doctor, we're federal..."

She cut him off mid-sentence. "The government has no relevance to our business here." A subtle movement of her head put the tall men into motion. They handled the intruders out of the room in half a minute of sullen shuffling, and the unit was restored to its research mission. As the door closed she addressed her volunteers:

"Gentlemen, to bed!" The slippered feet of the guinea pigs filed quickly by the doctor and into the sleeping area. A few gave utterance to their respect as they passed.

"Way to go, Dr. B!"

"Cool!"

"They're goin' home to Momma now!"

She nodded and smiled in response to these compliments, but watched for one particular face in the line of men. As Hank drew near to her, she raised an eyebrow, cast a sharp look at him, and asked, "Well? What's all this?"

"Doctor B," he asked, "if I knew half as much as everyone thinks I know, and if I could foresee strange catastrophes, why then, I ask you, would I need to do drug studies?"

She shrugged, and all the men lay down to offer up their blood to the beautiful doctor and her elves. As the tubes were filled with crimson fluid and clinked into their neat metal racks, the catheters were removed from veins and thrown into bright red trash can liners, and the last few droplets were daubed up into cotton filter-cloths, then the evening sun made its final, boiling reflection against the tall buildings in the distance, and the guinea pigs closed their eyes and slipped into a dream.

Bildad

Terrors frighten them on every side,
and chase them at their heels,
Disaster is hungry for them,
and calamity is ready for their stumbling.
By disease their skin is consumed,
Death the Firstborn, consumes their limbs.
—Job 18:11-13

The dauntful cavy was Bildad the Shoe-Height.
If we took him out of his cage
he would weep and quiver and jerk,
literally scared shitless;
if we set him on the floor
he'd seek refuge under the most immediate furniture and
cower there.

Bildad had few adventures in his short life.
One day he went to school and cringed at the children.
One month while we were away
he summered in the wilds of Northeast Philly,
where he ate watermelon
and cowered under a lawn chair on real grass.

And the lord smote Bildad with boils,
and an abcess on his neck came open
spewing blood and pus.
He screamed and shat with terror at the vet's.
The vet said the infection would go to his brain.

And then a strange thing happened:
Bildad the Shoe-Height forgat to be afraid.
He became an intrepid explorer.

Each day as his walk grew crazier
he doggedly lurched and sidled and swam,
penetrating ever deeper into the house,
yea unto the farthest reaches of the back bedroom.

Then one morning
he lay chill and trusting on my lap;
we said a long goodbye.
Half an hour later he was dead,
gone to that land where none have need
ever to cower again.

We shrouded him in a plastic bag,
and entombed him in the freezer.
Our daughter viewed him daily for a month,
after which Daddy took him to his lab
in a tote-bag hearse, with straphanger cortege,
and Bildad the Shoe-Height's mortal remains
joined those of all the other guinea pigs
and plunged skyward
in a shaft of transmogrifying fire.

—*ESTHER GREENLEAF MÜRER* (1996)

The Baby
BY OCTAVE MIRBEAU
Translated from the French by Robert Helms

"L'Enfant" originally appeared in the Paris periodical *La France* on October 21, 1885.

Motteau gave his testimony as follows:

"There you have it, your honor. You've listened to all these people—my good neighbors and my good friends. They haven't cut me any slack, and that's fair enough. They felt uncomfortable as long as I was in Boulaie-Blanche, and as long as there were no cops between them and the barrels of my shotgun. They may not like me, of course, but they're careful not to let their hatred show, because they know that Motteau is not someone to be played with. Today, it's a different story. See? I shrug my shoulders and I laugh in spite of myself.

"Maheu—one-eyed Maheu, who's come to tell you that I'm a murderer and a thief—OK, fine! It was Maheu that, last year at the Gravoir Auction, killed Blandé's guard. I was with you, you hoodlum, I don't deny it. And Léger, the hunchback who was churning out hypocrisies a minute ago—Léger robbed the church of Pontillou six months ago. Oh, he won't have the balls to deny it. We pulled that one off together, ain't that right, Léger?

"You don't know, do you, your honor, who it was that wrung the neck of Monsieur Jacquinot, that night when he was coming home from the Feuillet Fair? You've thrown a lot of innocent people in jail for that one, after your endless investigations. It's Sorel—Sorel who demanded my head a moment ago, OK? What? Ain't you gonna protest, comrade? There's no way he can, don't you see? While he strangled the old guy, I went through his

237

pockets—ha! This surprises you? But look at them! We're not proud anymore, are we, boys? We're not arrogant. We're turning pale, we're shaking, and we're saying to ourselves that when we turn in Motteau for the same thing we want to clear ourselves of, we're just turning ourselves in, and the same guillotine is going to cut through all of our necks.

"Your honor, what I'm telling you is the truth, and you can believe me. We're all like this in Boulaie-Blanche. Blessed Mother! You better believe it! For two leagues, all around the hamlet, there's nothing but heather and gorse bushes on the one side, and nothing but sand and rocks on the other. Here and there are some thin little birch trees, and then of course plenty of those stunted pines that can't really grow. The cabbages, even—they won't come up in our gardens! The place is cursed. How do you expect us to live in it? Oh, there's the Bureau of Charity, isn't there? Come on—it's just a cute little joke. It gives nothing, or, it gives you nothing unless you're rich. And so, since we're not far from the woods, we begin by doing some poaching. Sometimes this brings in something, but then there's the dead season, and there's the guards who'll track you down, and trials, and jail. My God, jail! Here we go again! We're fed, then we build traps while we're waiting to get out. I ask you, judge, what would you do in our place? Would you work somewhere else? Go and get a job on a farm? The problem is, when we say we're from Boulaie-Blanche, it's as though we'd just come in from hell. They run us out of there with their pitch forks. So we've got to steal! And when someone makes up his mind to steal, he must decide to kill. The one thing doesn't go without the other. If I tell you everything here today, it's because you've got to know what's what in Boulaie-Blanche, and that the fault really lies with the authorities, who never bother to do anything for us, and who isolate us from life like mad dogs, or as if we had the plague.

"Now I'll get to the present business.

"I got married just about a year ago, and my wife got pregnant in the first month. I gave it some thought: a baby to feed, when we can't even feed ourselves—it's stupid. 'We have to make it disappear!' I told my wife. Fortunately, close to our place there's an old woman who wanders around, and she's good at working out schemes like this. In return for a hare and two rabbits that I gave her, she brought my wife some plants and then some powders that she put together to make—I don't know what concoction to drink. This didn't do a thing. Nothing. The old hobo lady told us, 'Don't worry yourselves: it's as good as dead. I tell you it'll come out dead.' Since she had a reputation around the neighborhood for being a sorceress who knows her stuff, I didn't concern myself any further. I said to myself, 'That's good, then. It'll come out dead.' But she lied, the old thief, as you'll see in a minute.

"One night, under a beautiful moon, I killed me a roe deer. I was coming back with the deer on my back, and I was all happy, because you just about never get a deer, on any night. It was around three in the morning when I got back to my place. There was a light in the window. This surprised me, so I beat on the door, which is always barricaded from inside when I'm not around. It didn't open. I knocked some more, a little harder. Then I heard this little crying and some cursing, and then a sort of dragging step that went across the tiles. And what do I see? My wife is half naked, pale as a corpse, and all splashed with blood. First I thought that somebody'd tried to kill her, but she said to me, 'Not so much noise, idiot! Can't you see I'm havin' the baby?' Holy shit! It had to come one of these days, but then when it did come, I was caught completely off guard. I came in, threw the deer in a corner, and hung my shotgun on a nail."

"'Did it come out dead at least?' I asked my wife.

"'Oh, yeah, dead—just take a look!' she says to me, and I see on the bed, in a bunch of bloody rags, some naked thing wiggling around.

"I looked at my wife, she looked at me, and for five minutes or so we were quiet.

"'Were you cryin'?' I asked her.

"'No!'

"'Did you hear somebody prowlin' around outside?'

"'No!'

"'Why'd you have the light on?'

"'It wasn't two minutes the candle was lit, before you knocked,' she told me.

"'All right,' I said. Then I grabbed the baby by the feet, and real quick, like we do with rabbits, I gave it a good belt in the head. After that I stuck it in my game bag and I got my shotgun down again. You can believe me if you want, yer honor, but I swear, through the whole thing I never even knew if it was a girl or a boy.

"I went to the Grand Pierre spring. All around, as far as you can see, there was nothing but some scattered heather, growing in between the piles of rocks. Not a tree or a house stood nearby, not even a path that led to the place! As for living creatures, you'll only see some shepherds and their sheep grazing up there when there's no more grass down in the fields. Right by the spring there's a deep clay quarry that's been abandoned for a few hundred years. Some undergrowth hides the open mouth of the pit from your eye. That's where I go to hide my gun, and to hide myself when the cops are payin' me a visit. Who would dare to venture into that deserted place, which people seriously believe is haunted by ghosts? Nothing to fear. I threw the baby in the quarry, and I heard the sound of it hitting the bottom: 'Plunk!' Daylight was breaking, very pale, behind the hill.

"Coming back, in the path from Boulaie-Blanche, I spotted a gray form behind the hedge, something like the back of a man or a wolf—you can't always make things out so well, in the half-light, even if you do it all the time. It was sliding softly, crouching down low, creeping along, and it stopped.

"'Hey!' I yelled in a loud voice. 'If you're a man, show yourself or I'll shoot!'

"'Look, Motteau, it's me!' said the form, standing up all of a sudden.

"'Yeah, it's me,' I said, 'and don't forget, Maheu, there's a load of buckshot in my gun for nosy people.'

"And he says, 'Oh, no problem! I'm resetting my traps. But you know... it's not only the deer that squeal when you kill them.'

"'No!' I told him, 'There's also chicken-shits like you, you ugly one-eyed fuck!' I aimed at him, but I didn't shoot. I don't know why. I was wrong. Next day, Maheu went to get the cops.

"Now listen to me carefully, your honor. There are thirty households in Boulaie-Blanche: that's to say thirty women and thirty men. Have you counted how many living kids there are in those thirty households? There are only three. And the others—the suffocated ones, the strangled ones, the buried ones: in other words, the dead ones—have you counted them? Go and dig up the ground, down there in the skinny shadows of the birches, or at the feet of those scrawny pines. Drop a pole down into the wells. Turn over the gravel and sweep the sand away from the quarries. Under the birches and the pines, at the bottoms of the wells, mixed in with the sand and the pebbles, you'll see more bones of newborns than there are bones of men and women in the graveyards of the big cities. Go into the houses and ask the men, both young and old, what they've done with all the babies their wives

"All right! Maheu, you see that it's not just the deer that squeal when you kill them."

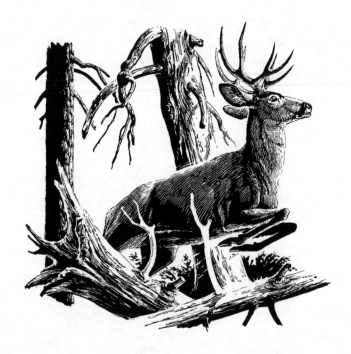

How You'll Know a Pro:
The Signs of a Professional Guinea Pig
BY ROBERT HELMS & ALISON LEWIS

Wears sweat pants, shirts, and wristwatches printed with the logos of research units.

Knows more about blood chemistry than a second-year medical student.

Is still wearing a patient name-bracelet from the study he was in yesterday.

Has tattoos commemorating diseases, like "I survived malaria @ NIH, Summer 1993."

Wears EKG electrodes from studies home on his body so his sweetie can chew them off.

Interrogates waitresses about the poppyseed content of bread products.

Holds casual conversations about his bilirubin levels. Gives unsolicited medical advice that works.

Refers to his anticubital vein as his "financial pipeline." Calls research units by the recruiter's name: "I'll see you down at Terry's place."

Pays off small debts with meal vouchers for hospital cafeterias.

Automatically reaches for a urine jug every time he uses his own toilet and mutters "mid-stream, clean-catch..."

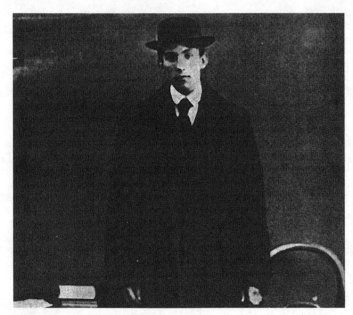

Plebeian Life is Cheap:
The Will Of Andre Soudy

Andre Soudy, a spice worker by trade, was guillotined in Paris on April 10, 1913 at age twenty. He had been a member of the then-famous Bonnot Gang, a group of anarchist-illegalists who robbed the rich and were the first to use an automobile as their means of escape from a crime scene. During the trial, he compared the working conditions in the spice mills to those in the plantations described in the American novel *Uncle Tom's Cabin*, and he also said, "If I'd had a situation befitting my intelligence, I would not have become an illegalist." On April 11, the Paris newspaper *l'Aurore* published the last will and testament of the newly executed man, which reads as follows:

La Sante Prison, April 17, 1913 This is my will:
Am I, Soudy, condemned to death by the representatives of so-called "Justice?"

WHEREAS it is my duty, and since I am expected to inform conscious and organized people of my final wishes,
FIRSTLY I bequeath to M. Etienne, the Minister of War, my crowbar, my squirrel monkeys, and my skeleton keys... to open the door of militarism;
SECONDLY to the Dean of the Faculty of Medicine, the hemispheres of my brain;
THIRDLY to the Museum of Anthropology, my skull, and I stipulate that it be placed on display to benefit the community soup kitchens;
FOURTHLY to the Barbers' Union and to all conscious, alcoholic workers, my hair, which shall be placed on public sale to benefit the cause, and for solidarity;
FIFTHLY and lastly, I bequeath to Anarchism my autograph, so that the apostles and the clowns of that powerful philosophy can use it to serve their cynical individualism.

Soudy.

Andre's family claimed the body and he was anonymously buried at the municipal cemetery in his home town, Beaugency (Loiret), France. The law prohibited marking the grave of an executed criminal. In spite of the above will, no autopsy was performed and he was left in his basic two pieces. The bodies of his two guillotine-buddies and former partners, however, were not claimed, and their cadavers went straight to the Faculty of Medicine. One of these was Raymond Callemin, called "Ray the Scientist" by his friends. It was made public that Callemin's nervous and vascular systems were in good condition, that there was no pathological defect in his brain, and that his brain was of normal weight.

-ROBERT HELMS

About the Creator of Guinea Pig Zero:

Robert Helms has been volunteering the use of his healthy body for medical experiments since 1995. He is a self-taught historian who has worked as a house painter, a factory hand, a helper of mentally retarded adults, and a union organizer. As editor and publisher of the zine *Guinea Pig Zero*, he has appeared in the national media as a voice for human research subjects. In 1997 he was sued for libel for his criticisms of a research unit near his home in Philadelphia. Helms also writes about the early anarchist movement of that city.

Choose from today's most renowned international authors—every one an eventful addition to your personal library:

Best of Temp Slave! edited by Jeff Kelly
"The temps, in their own words, let us know what it is all about. Let's not kid ourselves. Temp is a euphemism for day laborer. George and Lennie are no longer merely ranch hands. They work in law firms, banks, insurance companies and in your own workplace."
—Studs Terkel

Ivan Petrov: Russia through a Shot Glass by C.S. Walton
"Ivan Petrov is a potent brew—part roaring Rabelaisian tale and part social case study, with a dash of existential rebellion."
—William Brumfield, author of *Lost Russia*

A Terrible Thunder: The Story of the New Orleans Sniper by Peter Hernon
"A Terrible Thunder is more than just another fashionable journalistic rehashing of a crime. In its depiction of Essex's abrupt transmogrification it raises questions about the accumulated effect of petty but persistent injustices and about the individual's capacity to endure aggrievement."
—Mell Watkins, *New York Times*

Little Tenement on the Volga by C.S. Walton
"Maintaining a detailed, personal view, Walton captures much that's vividabout the hardships, ironies, and small victories of life in the far-flungterritories of contemporary Russia."
—Kirkus Reviews

A Letter To, For and About Mom, Dad and I by Cory Kapczynski

(order online @ www.gcpress.com)